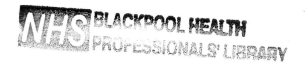
MRCS Picture Questions

Book 3

MRCS Picture Questions

Book 3

Edited by

Tjun Tang MD MRCS
Specialist Registrar in General & Vascular Surgery
Eastern Deanery, UK

Adrian Harris MD FRCSEd (GenSurg)
Consultant Upper GI & Laparoscopic Surgeon
Hinchingbrooke NHS Trust Hospital, Huntingdon, UK

Senthil Nachimuthu MS MRCSEd
Clinical Fellow in General Surgery
Hinchingbrooke NHS Trust Hospital, Huntingdon, UK

BV Praveen MS FRCS (Ed) FRCS (Eng) FRCS (Glas) FRCS (Ire) FRCS (Gen)
Consultant Colorectal Surgeon
Southend University Hospital
Honorary Clinical Senior Lecturer
Queen Mary University of London
Associate DME, Eastern Deanery
Examiner, Intercollegiate MRCS Examination

Foreword by
Pradip K Datta MS FRCS (Ed) FRCS (Eng) FRCS (Ire) FRCS (Glas)
Senior Examiner and Council Member
The Royal College of Surgeons of Edinburgh

Radcliffe Publishing
Oxford • New York

Radcliffe Publishing Ltd
18 Marcham Road
Abingdon
Oxon OX14 1AA
United Kingdom

www.radcliffe-oxford.com

Electronic catalogue and worldwide online ordering facility.

British Library Cataloguing in Publication Data

A catalogue record for this book is available from the British Library.

ISBN-13: 978 184619 108 4

Typeset by Pindar New Zealand (Egan Reid), Auckland, New Zealand
Printed and bound by Konway Printhouse, Penang, Malaysia

Contents

Foreword

It gives me great pleasure to write a foreword to the third volume in this series, not least because I have known Mr Praveen ever since his pre-Fellowship days shortly after he came to the UK in the early 1990s. Now, as a Consultant Surgeon in Southend, he has established himself as a good, enthusiastic and committed surgical teacher.

In this day and age surgical teachers are a rare breed. If one was to 'triage' the responsibilities of a surgeon in the NHS, teaching would end up pretty low in the order of priorities – first comes service provision (and quite rightly too), then 'number crunching' of patients treated to keep managers happy, private practice, research and family. Praveen has been able to strike a superb balance with considerable emphasis on teaching. This book is the outcome of the painstaking collection of clinical material over many years by the editors, aided by colleagues who have contributed much towards this very worthwhile publication.

Surgical trainees sometimes go from pillar to post in search of good teaching. The MRCS trainees should consider themselves lucky to have this book to prepare for the examination. As an examiner for the MRCS, I can assure the reader that this book comprehensively covers every aspect of Surgery in General including pathology, and answers all questions that can conceivably be asked either in the MCQs or Final Assessment. Some of the material is in such fine detail that I dare say the book would also be useful for the Higher Surgical Trainee preparing for the Exit FRCS examination.

As a person in the autumn of his surgical career, it gives me immense personal pleasure to see this publication come to fruition – edited by very committed young teachers, ably supported by several consultants and up and coming young surgeons who are setting out on the road to a surgical vocation. 'A picture is equal to a thousand words' – this adage is exemplified by the excellent pictures in this volume generously contributed by many young surgeons.

In writing this foreword, I must be careful not to stray into making it a 'book review'; that must be somebody else's job. All I can say is that the reader will find the following pages a compelling read. The quality of authorship is such that I will be surprised if other books did not soon emerge from the same stable. I wish the authors every success.

Pradip K Datta
MS FRCS (Ed) FRCS (Eng) FRCS (Ire) FRCS (Glasg)
Senior Examiner and Council Member
The Royal College of Surgeons of Edinburgh
September 2009

Preface

It gives us great pleasure to present our book to you. It is designed for candidates sitting both the new intercollegiate MRCS examination as well as the undergraduate clinical examinations in surgery. The method of presentation and topics are drawn from our own experiences during preparation for our examinations. The book provides visual revision material to reinforce core subject matter. The questions are based around a photograph or a set of pictures with each question slightly more difficult than the previous one.

With the new European Working Time Directive and the reduction in doctors' hours, trainees may find it more difficult to be exposed to all the different clinical cases. The MRCS examination requires candidates to acquire knowledge of the presentation and appearance of a wide range of surgical problems and we believe this book will assist students and trainees to acquire useful packages of information, not only for examination purposes but also to help them during their clinical practice. The combination of clinical photos and questions is perhaps the best way to revise both the clinical aspects and the subject matter associated with them. It is also believed that seeing clinical cases and reading about them at the same time, reinforces knowledge retention.

Case selection is based not only upon the editors' experiences but also those of other distinguished clinicians in different subspecialties. All contributors have been through the rigours of the MRCS examination and several are current intercollegiate MRCS examiners. Typical examination subject material and questions are presented.

We hope you enjoy working your way through this picture book and please do let us have your valued comments. We wish you all the best in your examinations and surgical career.

TT, AH, SN and BVP
September 2009

'The conditions necessary for the surgeon are four: first, he should be learned; second, he should be expert; third, he must be ingenious; and fourth, he should learn to adapt himself.'

Guy de Chauliac, 1300–68

List of contributors

MAJOR CONTRIBUTORS

Sections 1 and 2

Mr Szabolcs Gergely
Consultant Upper GI and Laparoscopic Surgeon
Hinchingbrooke NHS Trust Hospital,
*   Huntingdon*

Section 4

Mr Natarajan Sezhian
Consultant Urologist
James Paget NHS Trust Hospital, Great
*   Yarmouth*

Mr CJ Shukla
Specialist Registrar (Urology)
Norfolk & Norwich University Teaching
*   Hospital, Norfolk*

Dr Min Yen Wong
Specialist Registrar (Radiology)
Norfolk & Norwich University Hospital,
*   Norfolk*

CONTRIBUTORS

Mr Vamsi Velchuru
Clinical Fellow (General Surgery)
James Paget NHS Trust Hospital, Great
*   Yarmouth*

Mr Gerald David
Clinical Fellow (General Surgery)
Mid Cheshire Hospitals NHS Foundation Trust,
*   Crewe*

Dr Iain Au-Yong
Specialist Registrar (Radiology)
Nottingham Rotation

Acknowledgements

Medical Photography Services
James Paget NHS Trust Hospital, Great Yarmouth

Medical Illustration Department
Southend NHS Trust Hospital, Essex

Department of Radiology
Southend NHS Trust Hospital, Essex

Mr Ashley Brown
Former Clinical Tutor and Consultant Surgeon(Retd)
Southend NHS Trust Hospital, Essex

Alphonse Tadross
Associate Specialist (General Surgery)
James Paget NHS Trust Hospital, Great Yarmouth

Dedications

Tjun Tang: 'To my wife Nicole, for her love, patience and understanding and to my wonderful parents for their never-ending support and love over the years.'

Adrian Harris: 'To my wife Fiona, for her love and understanding; to my children Anna, Rachel and Kirsten, who bring us such joy; and to my brother Tim, who is never far away.'

Senthil Nachimuthu: 'To my patients and teachers from whom I am learning surgery, and to my parents and colleagues for their guidance and support all along.'

BV Praveen: 'To my wife Nandini, for her patience and understanding; to my daughter, Prakruti, who has brought us such joy.'

Section 1

Laparoscopic surgery

Case 1

The following pictures demonstrate the initial approach to a laparoscopic operation.

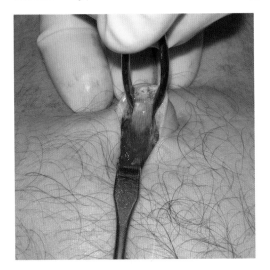

Figure 1.1a

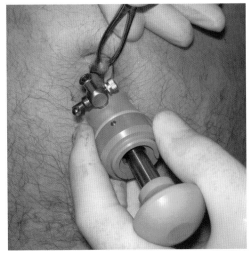

Figure 1.1c

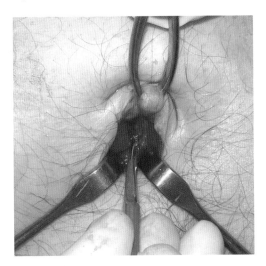

Figure 1.1b

Questions

Q1 Which technique for access to create a pneumoperitoneum is shown in Figures 1.1a–c?

Q2 Which anatomical structures need to be identified when applying it?

Q3 What alternative technique was widely used before this access?

Answers

(A1) The Hasson, or 'modified' Hasson technique.

(A2) The umbilicus and its insertion into the linea alba. The incision is made at this point, and the peritoneum punctured under direct vision to gain intraperitoneal access. A blunt trocar is then inserted and the abdomen insufflated with CO_2 under direct vision.

(A3) The Veress needle puncture. This is still used in some centres but concern has been raised over its technique of 'blind' puncture, which can result in increased risk of bowel or vascular trauma.

Case 2

Figure 1.2 shows part of a stack used in laparoscopic surgery, the 'endoflator'. It is important to know how this equipment works.

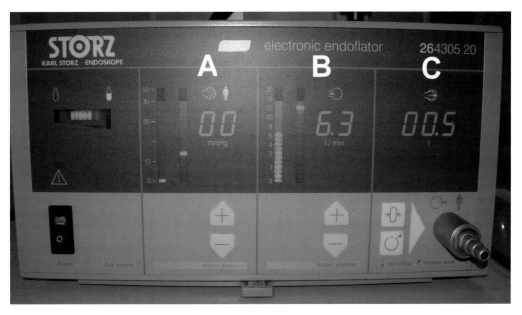

Figure 1.2

Questions

Q1 Describe the function of each of the columns labelled A, B, C.

Q2 What does the display to the left of 'A' indicate?

Q3 What might cause the left-hand LED in 'A' to rise sharply during surgery?

Answers

(A1) This unit controls CO_2 insufflation. 'A' indicates the pressure level within the abdomen and allows the constant pressure to be set at a particular limit. Here it is set at 12 mmHg (right-hand LED). The actual abdominal pressure is indicated by the left-hand LED, zero at present as the unit is disconnected. 'B' indicates gas flow rate, usually set at 6–10 Litres/minute. Once the abdomen has reached its preset pressure the flow rate falls to zero. When gas escapes, reducing the pressure, this is detected by the unit and the flow restarts. 'C' indicates the total amount of gas used.

(A2) This shows how much gas remains in the cylinder, and turns red when it is running low.

(A3) A sudden rise would be accompanied by an alarm signal, and indicates a sudden rise in the intra-abdominal pressure. A common cause of this is the patient beginning to wake up with the return of voluntary abdominal wall contraction (this is often an earlier 'warning signal' for the anaesthetist than the anaesthetic machine responses!). It may also happen with a mechanical block to the gas pipe (e.g. the tap is turned off).

Case 3

A diagnostic laparoscopy was undertaken for acute-onset right upper abdominal pain in a 17-year-old female patient. The ultrasound scan was normal.

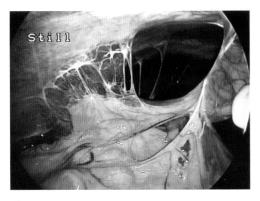

Figure 1.3

Questions

Q1 Figure 1.3 shows the view towards the right lobe of the liver. What pathology is shown on the picture?

Q2 What underlying disease is likely to have caused it?

Q3 What risks are associated with this condition?

Q4 What is the appropriate management for this patient?

Answers

(A1) This is Curtis–Fitz-Hugh syndrome. Adhesions develop between the liver and peritoneum following perihepatitis.

(A2) Chlamydia infection.

(A3) In cases with acute infective salpingitis, the risk of infertility may be higher than 50%.

(A4) Gynaecological referral; high vaginal swabs for microbiology to confirm diagnosis; antibiotics (doxycycline); infertility counselling.

Case 4

A diagnostic laparoscopy was undertaken to investigate intermittent abdominal pain in a young female. All other investigations were normal.

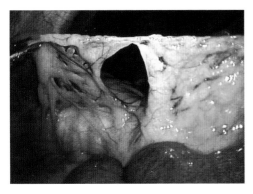

Figure 1.4

Questions

Q1 What pathology is visible on the picture?

Q2 What is the management?

Q3 What other conditions cause a similar clinical presentation?

Answers

(A1) A trans-omental defect.

(A2) This is large enough to cause subacute obstruction by trapping loops of small bowel. Treatment comprises simple division of the edge of the defect.

(A3) Any cause of bowel obstruction; in this age group, usually postoperative (e.g. appendicectomy) or congenital (e.g. Meckel's diverticular band) adhesions.

Case 5

This diagnostic laparoscopy was undertaken for recent, sudden-onset, constant increasing pain in a 20-year-old female patient. Ultrasound of pelvis was normal. Blood tests revealed a raised white count and CRP. Pregnancy test was negative.

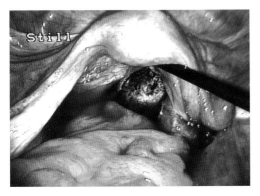

Figure 1.5

Questions

Q1 What abnormality is seen in the pelvis?

Q2 What is the cause?

Q3 How would you treat this condition?

Answers

(A1) A necrotic lesion in the right pelvis.

(A2) Torsion of an ovarian cyst.

(A3) Right salpingo-oophorectomy.

Case 6

Figure 1.6 shows the dissection of Calot's triangle during an elective laparoscopic cholecystectomy.

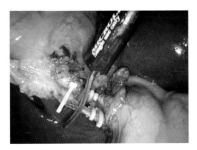

Figure 1.6

Questions

Q1 How is Calot's triangle defined?

Q2 What is the importance of Calot's triangle?

Q3 In Figure 1.6, what structures have been clipped and which one is about to be divided?

TV07635

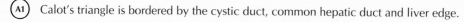

Answers

(A1)   Calot's triangle is bordered by the cystic duct, common hepatic duct and liver edge.

(A2)   It is an important anatomical entity as it clarifies the relationship between the biliary and vascular anatomy; the cystic artery usually runs across the triangle (i.e. behind the cystic duct) to the gallbladder. However, care must always be taken to dissect both cystic duct and artery before clipping and dividing tubular structures, which may not be what they seem. This is an area where anatomical anomalies are often seen; the 'normal' must be appreciated in order to discern the 'abnormal' and prevent serious bile duct injury.

(A3)   The cystic duct and artery have both been clipped, twice proximally and once distally. The artery is about to be divided. It usually lies posterior to the cystic duct, but vascular anatomy in this region can vary and occasionally the artery is anterior, as in this case.

Case 7

This 65-year-old male patient was admitted acutely with right upper quadrant pain, swinging pyrexia, raised white count and C-reactive protein (CRP).

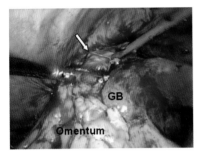

Figure 1.7

Questions

Q1 What is the condition being dealt with? What is indicated by the white arrow and what has caused this?

Q2 What are the most common diseases resulting in this type of problem?

Q3 What further investigations can be done to identify the cause intra/postoperatively?

Answers

A1 Subphrenic abscess. The arrow indicates the abscess cavity, which has been caused by perforation of a gallbladder empyema. Gallstone obstruction at the neck of the gallbladder caused a mucocoele which became infected, resulting in empyema. This then perforated causing omental adhesion, but the pus was not contained and leaked into the subphrenic space where it walled off as an abscess.

A2 Perforation of any abdominal viscus; liver abscess; basal pneumonia.

A3 On-table cholangiogram; intraoperative laparoscopic ultrasound.

Case 8

This 60-year-old female diabetic patient was admitted to the medical unit with a right lower lobe pneumonia and right upper abdominal pain. An ultrasound scan was performed on day three of her admission when she was not improving on antibiotics. It showed a distended thick-walled gallbladder with some gallstones within.

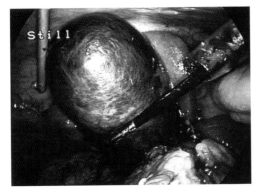

Figure 1.8

Questions

Q1 Describe the pathology on the picture.

Q2 Describe the role of percutaneous drainage alone in the management of this condition.

Q3 What condition other than gallstone cholecystitis can lead to this pathology?

Answers

(A1) A distended, thick-walled, gangrenous gallbladder.

(A2) Despite co-morbidities, there is no place for radiological drainage in this case. The cause of the problem is an obstructed gallbladder, which has become necrotic due to increased tissue pressure causing localised ischaemia. The only treatment is surgery.

(A3) Occasionally this condition is seen in patients following major trauma or sepsis, in whom acalculous cholecystitis can develop.

Case 9

Figure 1.9 depicts a view at the start of a routine laparoscopic cholecystectomy.

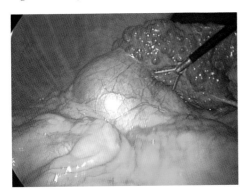

Figure 1.9

Questions

(Q1) What is the liver abnormality shown in this picture?

(Q2) What are the increased risks when performing surgery for a patient having this condition?

(Q3) What are the complications that develop due to the increased transhepatic venous pressure gradient?

(Q4) What interventional/surgical procedures do you know that deal with these complications?

Answers

(A1) Cirrhosis.

(A2) Persistent bleeding due to inadequate production of clotting factors. Also the liver may be less supple and gallbladder retraction may therefore be restricted, causing difficult access to Calot's triangle.

(A3) Oesophageal and gastric varices, which may bleed.

(A4) Surgical shunts have been previously described, but most have an unacceptably high risk of complications or side effects. Currently the best treatment is TIPSS (Transjugular Intrahepatic Porto–Systemic Shunt).

Case 10

During the dissection of Calot's triangle in a routine laparoscopic cholecystectomy, the following anatomy is encountered:

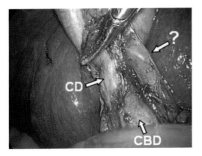

Figure 1.10

Questions

Q1   The cystic duct (CD) and common bile duct (CBD) have been identified. What is the unknown structure?

Q2   How would you proceed at this point?

Q3   If you think this is the cystic artery, what can you do to make sure you don't divide the wrong structure?

Answers

(A1)   This is an aberrant right hepatic artery (RHA), looping up with retraction of the gallbladder before plunging back into the right lobe of liver.

(A2)   Slowly and carefully, and call your consultant! Further dissection of this structure revealed the cystic artery as a much smaller branch coming off the apex of the loop. In fact, with experience, this is unlikely to be clipped in error because it is just too big to be the cystic artery, but that only applies if this anatomical variation is considered when operating.

(A3)   Pull the camera back to obtain a wide view of the liver, and then gently occlude the lumen of this structure with atraumatic graspers. If it is the RHA, the whole liver lobe will become noticeably paler than the left lobe. If in doubt, don't cut it. The cystic artery is confirmed by ensuring it ends in the gallbladder and is clipped as close to the gallbladder as possible.

Case 11

These images were obtained intraoperatively during four different laparoscopic cholecystectomies.

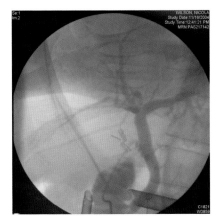

Figure 1.11a

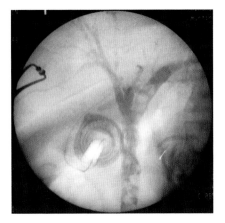

Figure 1.11c

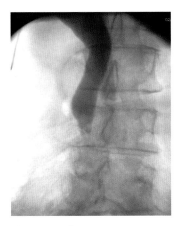

Figure 1.11b

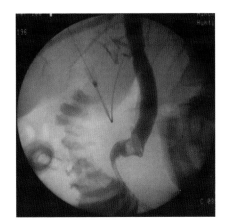

Figure 1.11d

Questions

(Q1) What imaging test has been performed?

(Q2) What needs to be assessed in the interpretation of these tests?

(Q3) Describe the findings in Figures 1.11a–d.

Answers

(A1)   Intraoperative cholangiogram.

(A2)   It is vital to know how to interpret these images in order not to miss significant pathology. The easiest way to view a cholangiogram is AFF – Anatomy, Filling defects, and Flow of contrast. Anatomy should assess a normal tapered distal CBD, size of duct (dilated?) and biliary tree, with appropriate spread of intrahepatic branches. Filling defects are stones, although occasionally a bubble of air can mimic a stone. And the contrast should flow rapidly into the duodenum.

(A3)   Figure 1.11a – Normal cholangiogram.

Figure 1.11b – Dilated CBD with several small stones obstructing the ampulla.

Figure 1.11c – Dilated intra- and extrahepatic biliary tree with multiple stones in CBD, common hepatic duct and left hepatic duct.

Figure 1.11d – Dilated CBD with stones in distal duct sitting in the upper pigtail of a biliary stent.

Case 12

This image was obtained preoperatively.

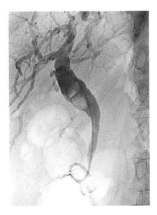

Figure 1.12

Questions

Q1 What diagnostic test has been performed?

Q2 Describe the abnormalities evident in this picture.

Q3 What are the treatment options?

Answers

(A1) ERCP (Endoscopic Retrograde Cholangio Pancreatography) with insertion of pigtail stent.

(A2) Dilated proximal CBD with two large stones causing obstruction. Dilatation of intrahepatic biliary tree.

(A3) It appears that the ERCP has failed to remove the stones as a stent has been inserted. Reasons for failed ERCP include stones that are large, impacted and multiple; ampullary anomalies (duodenal diverticulum, ampullary stricture); and previous gastric surgery. Laparoscopic CBD exploration is the optimal treatment, and in this case successfully cleared the duct without complication.

Case 13

In this patient, common bile duct stones were found on intraoperative cholangiogram.

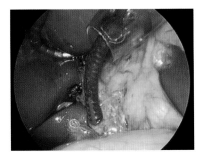

Figure 1.13a

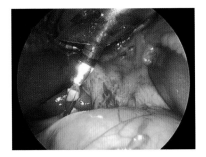

Figure 1.13b

Questions

(Q1)   What procedure is being carried out in Figure 1.13a?

(Q2)   What other technique is available to access the CBD and what are its advantages/disadvantages?

(Q3)   What technique is being demonstrated in Figure 1.13b?

Answers

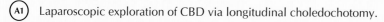 Laparoscopic exploration of CBD via longitudinal choledochotomy.

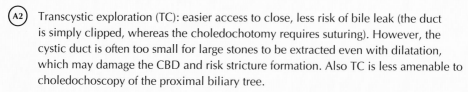 Transcystic exploration (TC): easier access to close, less risk of bile leak (the duct is simply clipped, whereas the choledochotomy requires suturing). However, the cystic duct is often too small for large stones to be extracted even with dilatation, which may damage the CBD and risk stricture formation. Also TC is less amenable to choledochoscopy of the proximal biliary tree.

(A3) Extraction of a stone using a Dormia basket.

Case 14

This patient underwent a laparoscopic cholecystectomy and exploration for CBD stones. The duct was successfully cleared laparoscopically.

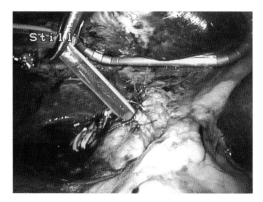

Figure 1.14a

Questions

Q1 What is shown in Figure 1.14a? What other precaution is required before finishing the operation?

Q2 What is the typical postoperative management?

Q3 What test is shown in Figure 1.14b, and what should be done after its successful completion?

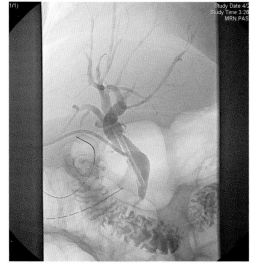

Figure 1.14b

Answers

(A1) Insertion of a T-tube. A drain must also be placed near to the CBD repair to drain off any bile that leaks in the immediate postoperative period. Most bile duct closures leak a little but as long as the duct has been cleared of distal obstruction, this will settle rapidly.

(A2) The drain is removed after 24–48 hours if patient is well and drainage minimal. The patient can go home with the T-tube in situ. A T-tube cholangiogram is arranged 2–3 weeks post-op.

(A3) This is a T-tube cholangiogram, showing normal biliary anatomy, no residual stones, and rapid contrast flow into duodenum. The T-tube can now be removed. The time delay in removal is to allow a fistula to form around the latex tube so that any residual bile flow after removal of the T-tube will drain out of the peritoneal cavity, thus minimising the risk of biliary peritonitis.

Case 15

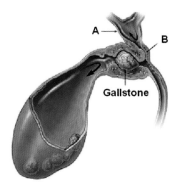

Figure 1.15

Questions

Q1 What condition is illustrated in Figure 1.15?

Q2 How is this condition classified?

Q3 How is the diagnosis made, and what are the initial and definitive treatments?

Answers

(A1) Mirizzi's syndrome.

(A2) Two categories: Type 1 (as in the figure) where a stone is stuck in the cystic duct or Hartmann's pouch. This causes inflammatory changes and external compression to the common hepatic duct (B), causing obstructive jaundice (A). In Type 2 the chronic inflammation progresses to form a fistula between the CD and CHD thus releasing the stone into the CHD/CBD. Type 2 is further subdivided according to the size of the fistula as a proportion of the CBD diameter (in thirds).

(A3) Diagnosis is by combination of USS (Ultrasound Scan) and MRCP or ERCP. Usually a stent is required in the short term to relieve obstruction. A laparoscopic cholecystectomy is then performed but often very difficult because of the degree of inflammation and fibrosis that has occurred. Typically a subtotal cholecystectomy is all that can be safely achieved.

Case 16

These pictures were all taken at diagnostic laparoscopy for suspected appendicitis.

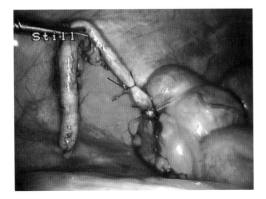

Figure 1.16a

Questions

Q1   Describe the steps involved in a typical appendicectomy.

Q2   What differences are evident between Figures 1.16a and 1.16b?

Q3   What is the diagnosis in Figure 1.16c and what postoperative treatment would you prescribe?

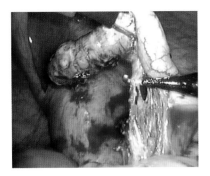

Figure 1.16b

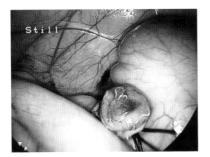

Figure 1.16c

Answers

(A1)   Division of the mesoappendix, clipping the appendicular artery; endoloops placed around the base of the appendix; division of the appendix and removal in a bag.

(A2)   Figure 1.16a shows a thin, mildly inflamed appendix; in Figure 1.16b, a gangrenous appendix tip is about to perforate (acute suppurative appendicitis).

(A3)   Threadworm. This can occasionally be a cause of appendicitis in the UK; when found, the worms on the stump should be cauterised carefully, and the patient (plus family) given a course of anti-helminth antibiotics, such as Mebendazole.

Case 17

Figures 1.17a and 1.17b were taken during two different laparoscopic hernia repairs.

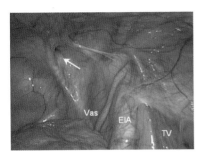

Figure 1.17a

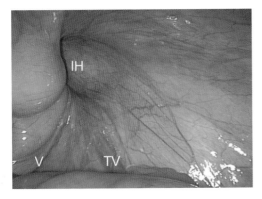

Figure 1.17b

Questions

(Q1) What is the diagnosis in each case?

(Q2) What approach has been undertaken to repair these hernias?

(Q3) Identify the anatomy as indicated by the abbreviations.

(Q4) Where precisely has the mesh been placed in Figure 1.17c and what are the principles guiding this placement?

(Q5) Figure 1.17d demonstrates a number of right-sided herniae seen at initial laparoscopy. Identify each labelled defect.

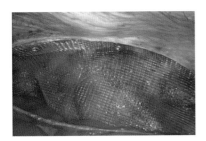

Figure 1.17c

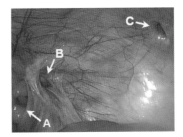

Figure 1.17d

Answers

(A1) Figure 1.17a: direct right inguinal hernia.
Figure 1.17b: indirect right inguinal hernia.

(A2) This is a TAPP repair (TransAbdominal PrePeritoneal).

(A3) Vas/V – vas deferens; EIA – external iliac artery; TV – testicular vessels.

(A4) The mesh is in the preperitoneal space. It should be big enough, usually 10 × 15 cm, to cover all potential weak spots (direct, indirect and femoral hernia sites) and reach the midline, as this is a common site of recurrence. Some surgeons fix it with tacks although there is evidence to show this may not be necessary. The peritoneum is closed over the mesh to prevent bowel adhesions.

(A5) A – Femoral; B – Indirect inguinal; C – Spigelian.

Case 18

These pictures relate to anti-reflux surgery for gastro-oesophageal reflux disease.

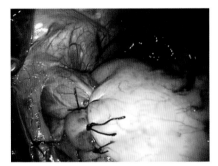

Figure 1.18a

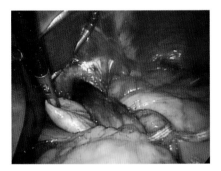

Figure 1.18b

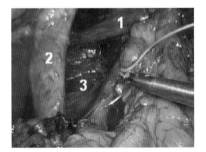

Figure 1.18c

Questions

Q1 Describe the general principles of anti-reflux surgery. What procedure has been completed in Figure 1.18a? What modifications to this operation can be employed?

Q2 Describe the phase of the operation depicted in Figure 1.18b.

Q3 Identify the numbered parts in Figure 1.18c. What phase of the operation is being carried out?

Answers

(A1) Reduction of the hiatus hernia; Crural repair; creation of a retro-oesophageal window; loose ('floppy') fundal wrap around the distal oesophagus. In Figure 1.18a, a Nissen 360° wrap has been performed. The wrap may be modified to a partial anterior ('Dor') or posterior ('Toupet') fundoplication.

(A2) This is called the 'shoeshine' step – to demonstrate both an adequate window through which the fundus will pass, and also adequate mobilisation of the fundus so that it will wrap without tension.

(A3) No. 1 – oesophagus; No. 2 – right crus; No. 3 – aorta. This is the crural repair, using '0' size Ethibond™ sutures.

Section 2

GI endoscopy

Case I

This view is seen on intubating the pharynx.

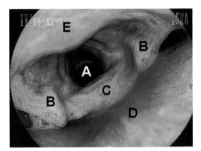

Figure 2.1

Questions

(Q1) Identify the labelled parts in Figure 2.1.

(Q2) Where should the tip of the endoscope be aimed to successfully intubate the oesophagus?

Answers

A1   A – trachea; B – arytenoid cartilage; C – transverse arytenoid muscle; D – posterior pharyngeal wall (hypopharynx); E – epiglottis.

A2   Between C and D.

Case 2

This patient has undergone an endoscopy for epigastric pain. The history includes arthritis for which the patient is taking painkillers.

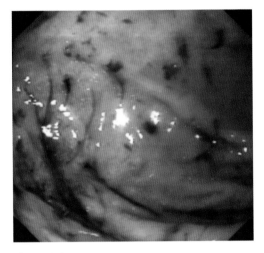

Figure 2.2

Questions

Q1 Describe the appearances in Figure 2.2.

Q2 What is the diagnosis and how would you treat this condition?

Answers

(A1)   Erythematous mucosa with erosions and haemorrhagic spots.

(A2)   Acute erosive gastritis. This is typical of NSAID gastropathy. Treatment comprises Proton Pump Inhibitor (PPI) treatment and CLO test with helicobacter eradication if positive, plus stopping all NSAID medication.

Case 3

This was an upper GI endoscopy performed to investigate symptoms of heartburn and dysphagia.

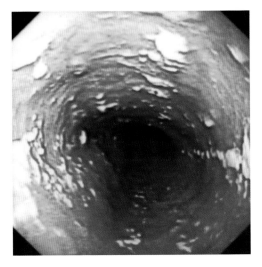

Figure 2.3

Questions

(Q1) Describe the clinical findings as shown in Figure 2.3.

(Q2) What is the diagnosis and how would you confirm it?

(Q3) How would you treat this patient?

(Q4) Which types of patient typically present like this?

Answers

(A1) Scattered multiple white plaques with erythematous mucosa.

(A2) Candida oesophagitis. Confirmed with microbiology swab/brushings +/- biopsy.

(A3) This is treated with an antifungal agent such as Fluconazole.

(A4) Immunocompromised, septic or postoperative patients after major surgery.

Case 4

These four pictures demonstrate increasing severity of the same condition.

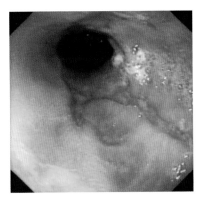

Figure 2.4a

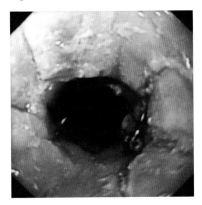

Figure 2.4b

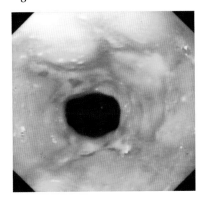

Figure 2.4c

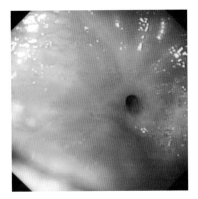

Figure 2.4d

Questions

(Q1) What is the diagnosis?

(Q2) How is this condition classified?

(Q3) What is the grade of severity in each case?

(Q4) How would you manage a case of severe ulcerative oesophagitis?

Answers

(A1) Reflux oesophagitis.

(A2) Savary-Miller classification, Grades 1–4:
Grade 1: Erosions in one mucosal fold
Grade 2: Erosions in several mucosal folds, the erosions may be confluent
Grade 3: Circumferential erosions in the distal oesophagus
Grade 4: Chronic complications such as ulcers, stenosis, or scarring with Barrett's
        metaplasia.

More recently the 'LA classification' has been suggested but this has not been widely adopted in the UK.

(A3) Figure 2.4a: Grade 2, Figure 2.4b: Grade 2, Figure 2.4c: Grade 3, Figure 2.4d: Grade 4.

(A4) Biopsies should be taken at the index endoscopy to exclude an occult ulcerating tumour. The patient should take full dose PPI for 6–8 weeks then undergo repeat endoscopy to assess healing. If the ulcer persists further biopsies must be taken to exclude a persisting occult neoplasm, even if the preliminary biopsies were negative.

Case 5

This picture was taken during endoscopy to investigate dysphagia.

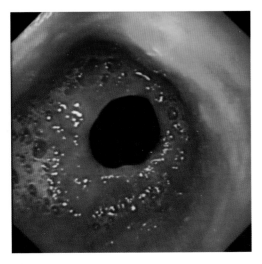

Figure 2.5

Questions

Q1 What is the condition?

Q2 What is the underlying cause?

Q3 How would you manage this patient?

Answers

(A1)   Peptic stricture of the oesophagus.

(A2)   Reflux oesophagitis.

(A3)   Biopsy to exclude malignancy, then proceed with endoscopic balloon dilatation.

Case 6

These two pictures demonstrate the same condition with different severity.

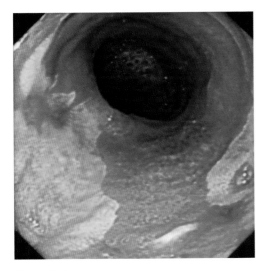

Figure 2.6a

Questions

(Q1) What is the condition?

(Q2) What treatment would you advise?

(Q3) How would you manage this patient in the long term?

(Q4) What advice would you give to the patient about the possible complications associated with this condition?

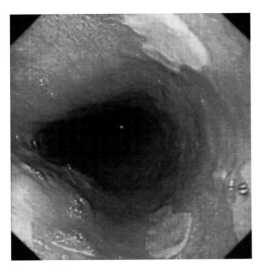

Figure 2.6b

Answers

(A1) Barrett's oesophagus.

(A2) Lifelong treatment with PPI should be advised. If symptoms are severe then anti-reflux surgery may be considered in some cases.

(A3) Regular endoscopy with 4-quadrant biopsies every 2 cm.

Without dysplasia: two-yearly endoscopy and biopsy.
Low-grade dysplasia: six-monthly histological surveillance.
High-grade dysplasia: consider surgery/endoscopic mucosal resection (EMR).

Most centres cease endoscopic surveillance beyond the age of 75 as the benefit outweighs the risks in this age group.

(A4) Untreated, this condition can lead to benign complications like ulceration and stricture. There is also a small but acknowledged risk of developing adenocarcinoma (cumulative risk of 0.8% per annum).

Case 7

These pictures were taken in different patients being investigated for dysphagia and weight loss.

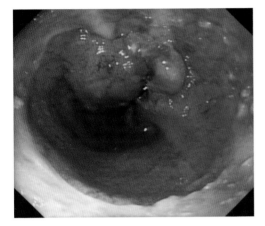

Figure 2.7a

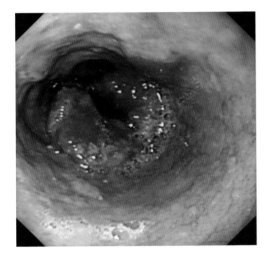

Figure 2.7b

Questions

(Q1)   What is the diagnosis?

(Q2)   How would you proceed with this endoscopy?

(Q3)   How would you manage this patient?

(Q4)   If this condition is inoperable, what other treatment options are available?

(Q5)   What are the two main histological subtypes of this condition and with what frequency do they currently present?

Answers

(A1) Oesophageal adenocarcinoma.

(A2) The patient requires multiple biopsies sent for urgent histology. The case should be referred to the local upper GI Multi-Disciplinary Team (MDT) without delay.

(A3) Staging CT (+/- staging laparoscopy if a junctional Type 2 or 3 tumour); MDT discussion regarding optimal treatment if operable – surgery with or without neoadjuvant chemotherapy.

(A4) Palliative chemo/radiotherapy, laser recanalisation or expandable metal stent.

(A5) Squamous cell and adenocarcinoma (rarely small cell). Historically the relative frequency was 90% squamous, 8% adenocarcinoma. However, over the past two to three decades there has been a gradual rise in the incidence of adenocarcinoma and concomitant decline in squamous carcinoma. This is thought to be due to multifactorial processes, including a combination of rise in obesity, hiatus hernia, acid reflux and resulting Barrett's oesophagus. The relative rates are now adenocarcinoma 60–70%, squamous 30–40%.

Case 8

This patient has been investigated and treated for dysphagia.

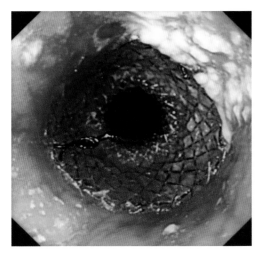

Figure 2.8

Questions

(Q1) What procedure has been undertaken?

(Q2) What other diagnosis can be made from this picture?

(Q3) What is the purpose of the knot seen in the 8 o'clock position?

Answers

(A1) Palliative stenting of an oesophageal tumour.

(A2) Candida oesophagitis.

(A3) Removal of the stent. This is sometimes required if the stent becomes displaced. However, stent removal can be hazardous, risking damage to the upper oesophagus or pharynx. The knot is grasped and the suture acts like a purse string, pulling the upper rim of the stent closed. It can then be more safely removed.

Case 9

This is the 'J' manoeuvre performed during a gastroscopy.

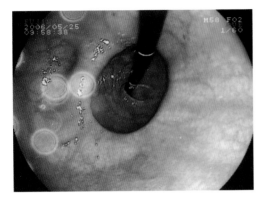

Figure 2.9

Questions

Q1 What abnormality is demonstrated in Figure 2.9?

Q2 What signs and symptoms can this condition cause?

Q3 What options are available to treat this condition?

Answers

(A1) This shows a large sliding hiatus hernia.

(A2) Typically heartburn, retrosternal discomfort and regurgitation, sometimes with quite significant volume. With excessive acid reflux patients may complain of a bad taste in the mouth and halitosis. Erosive etching of the teeth may be noticed by the dentist. Reflux can also be the cause of chronic cough or be misdiagnosed as 'asthma'.

(A3) Conservative: PPI plus lifestyle changes (avoid late meals and fizzy drinks, use raised pillow at night, weight loss, etc).

Surgical: anti-reflux procedures have a 90% chance of cure in patients who respond to PPIs. The hiatus hernia is repaired and the fundus wrapped loosely around the oesophagus. This may be a 360° Nissen procedure, or alternatively a partial wrap (posterior or anterior).

Case 10

These two gastroscopies were performed to investigate epigastric pain associated with melaena and hypotension.

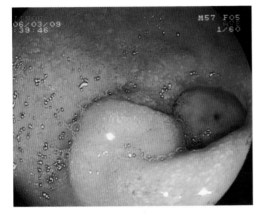

Figure 2.10a

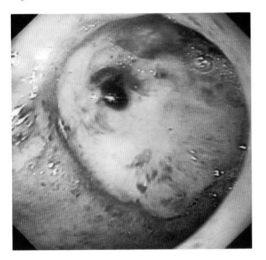

Figure 2.10b

Questions

Q1 What is the diagnosis?

Q2 In what precise location is the abnormality situated?

Q3 How would you proceed with this endoscopy?

Q4 What treatment would you advise for this patient?

Q5 What is the classification system for risk of re-bleed and what is the risk of re-bleed in this case?

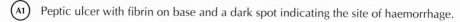

Answers

(A1) Peptic ulcer with fibrin on base and a dark spot indicating the site of haemorrhage.

(A2) Posterior wall of D2.

(A3) The base and circumference may be injected with 1:10000 adrenaline if oozing is seen. If dry, this ulcer may be left alone. A CLO test is performed to confirm helicobacter.

(A4) Treatment with HP eradication is recommended, as there is at least a 95% association between DU and helicobacter. Intravenous Omeprazole has been shown to reduce the risk of a re-bleed, and this is normally continued orally for a further six weeks. Usually, neither biopsy nor repeat endoscopy is required in DUs as these are only very rarely malignant. If the patient suffers a re-bleed, a second endoscopy is often done in theatre in case surgery is necessary.

(A5) Forrest levels 1–3:

Level	Stigmata	Risk of re-bleed
1a	Active arterial bleeding	55%
1b	Active non-pulsatile bleeding ('oozing')	30–50%
2a	Visible vessel	40%
2b	Adherent clot	20%
2c	Flat red or black spot	10%
3	Clean base	<5%

In these cases, classification is:
Figure 2.10a: Forrest 2c, 10% risk for re-bleed.
Figure 2.10b: Forrest 2b, 20% risk for re-bleed.

Case 11

This patient was admitted with hypertension and melaena. Initial endoscopy revealed a lot of blood in the stomach and no definite diagnosis was possible. The patient was resuscitated and a subsequent endoscopy showed this lesion.

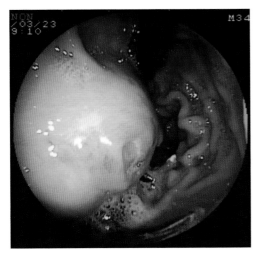

Questions

Q1 What is this lesion?

Q2 Describe its typical features.

Q3 How was the diagnosis confirmed?

Q4 How are these lesions classified with regard to prognosis?

Q5 How would you treat this patient?

Figure 2.11

Answers

(A1) A gastric GIST (GastroIntestinal Stromal Tumour).

(A2) Smooth subserosal lesion often with central ulceration.

(A3) Biopsy is only effective if deep enough to get a good sample of tissue. Positive c-kit staining (interstitial cells of Cajal, CD 34 and CD 117) is diagnostic for GIST. CT and endoluminal ultrasound (EUS) will confirm location, extent and evidence of metastatic disease.

(A4) They have a malignant potential, the extent of which depends on size of lesion and number of mitotic figures per HP field.

(A5) MDT discussion followed by local resection. Lymphadenectomy is not required. For recurrent and or metastatic disease, Glivec (imatinib mesylate, a tyrosine kinase inhibitor) may be used. For large tumours, Glivec is occasionally used preoperatively in an attempt to shrink the tumour.

Case 12

These two pictures demonstrate similar pathology. The patients were being investigated for epigastric pain, dysphagia and weight loss.

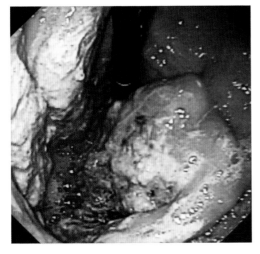

Figure 2.12a

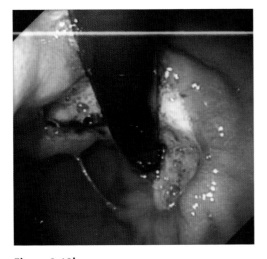

Figure 2.12b

Questions

- (Q1) What is the clinical diagnosis?
- (Q2) How would you confirm this?
- (Q3) How would you next manage this patient?
- (Q4) How are these lesions classified?
- (Q5) Upon what features does the prognosis depend?

Answers

(A1)   Carcinoma of the gastro-oesophageal junction.

(A2)   Multiple biopsies.

(A3)   Staging CT; MDT discussion; surgery +/- neoadjuvant chemotherapy if operable.

(A4)   Siewert classification, types I–III.
(I. Distal oesophagus, II. Junctional, III. Proximal gastric).

(A5)   TNM stage, histological subtypes, and age and co-morbidity of the patient.

Case 13

This is a view of a gastroscopy looking towards the antrum. The patient was being investigated for anaemia and weight loss.

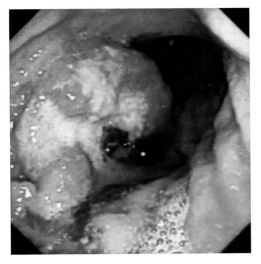

Figure 2.13

Questions

(Q1) What diagnosis is evident in this picture?

(Q2) Having staged the patient, if there are no contraindications what is the operation of choice?

(Q3) What are the main histological subtypes of this kind of lesion?

Answers

(A1)   Carcinoma of the stomach.

(A2)   Subtotal D2 gastrectomy.

(A3)   Adenocarcinoma, either intestinal or diffuse (otherwise known as 'linitis plastica').

Case 14

This picture demonstrates the 'J' view during a gastroscopy.

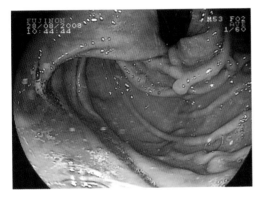

Figure 2.14

Questions

(Q1)   What feature does this picture demonstrate?

(Q2)   What other investigations may be useful in conjunction with endoscopy?

Answers

(A1) An intact fundoplication or 'wrap'. The clue is in the alignment of the proximal rugal folds. In the top left of the picture, vertical folds are seen passing up behind horizontal folds, which indicates the wrap is still intact.

(A2) This endoscopy has probably been done to investigate either prolonged dysphagia or recurrent reflux symptoms after a laparoscopic fundoplication. Other investigations which will be of help are repeat pH and manometry and a barium swallow/meal. These are important if reoperation is being considered.

Case 15

This picture was taken during a gastroscopy to investigate anaemia and weight loss.

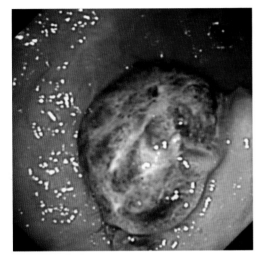

Figure 2.15

Questions

Q1   What is the diagnosis?

Q2   How would you further investigate this patient?

Q3   What is the treatment?

Q4   What is the prognosis of this condition?

Answers

(A1) Gastric melanoma.

(A2) Thorough examination to determine other melanotic lesions; CT chest, abdomen and pelvis.

(A3) If localised then R0 gastrectomy plus symptomatic control as required.

(A4) Poor: 9–12 months survival.

Case 16

This is a view of the distal oesophagus undertaken to investigate almost total dysphagia. The patient has no other significant co-morbidity other than Parkinson's disease.

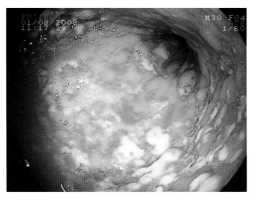

Figure 2.16

Questions

Q1 Describe the endoscopic findings.

Q2 Given that the endoscope passed easily into the stomach and 'J' manoeuvre revealed no junctional obstruction, what do you think is the diagnosis in this case?

Q3 What is the pathophysiology of this disease?

Q4 What treatment options are available for this patient?

Answers

(A1) Distal dilatation of the oesophagus, oesophagitis and food residue.

(A2) Achalasia.

(A3) Absence of the myoenteric (Auerbach) nerve plexus.

(A4) Endoscopic botulinum toxin injection – less effective, needs repeat injection.

Endoscopic balloon dilatation – can give good results but may need repeat dilatation, risk of perforation.

Surgical – Heller's myotomy (laparoscopic) – better long-term results; needs anterior wrap to prevent acid reflux after destruction of the lower oesophageal sphincter.

Case 17

This patient was undergoing endoscopic examination after recent emergency admission with left iliac fossa pain, raised temperature and white count, and small amount of PR bleeding.

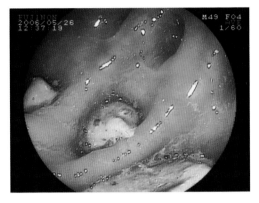

Figure 2.17

Questions

Q1 What examination is being carried out?

Q2 What is the diagnosis?

Q3 How is this managed in the acute setting?

Q4 How would you then manage this patient in the long term?

Answers

(A1) Flexible sigmoidoscopy/colonoscopy.

(A2) Diverticulosis/diverticulitis.

(A3) Conservative: bowel rest plus broad-spectrum antibiotics.

(A4) High-fibre diet; consider sigmoid colectomy if recurrent episodes.

Case 18

This picture was taken during investigation for altered bowel habit and weight loss.

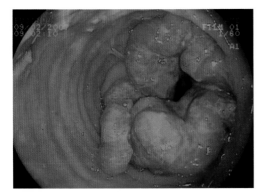

Figure 2.18

Questions

Q1   Describe the lesion.

Q2   What is the diagnosis?

Q3   How would you confirm this?

Q4   What further investigations are required, and what are the important factors to establish prior to treatment?

Q5   What are the treatment options for this patient?

Q6   What factors affect the choice of treatment?

Answers

(A1) Annular polypoid growth partially obstructing the lumen.

(A2) Carcinoma of the colon.

(A3) Multiple biopsies.

(A4) CT scan of the chest, abdomen and pelvis; TNM staging; presence or absence of metastases, synchronous lesions; fitness of patient for possible surgery.

(A5) Curative treatment:
- colectomy with or without adjuvant chemotherapy.

Palliative treatment:
- palliative resection/chemotherapy, defunctioning stoma or endoscopic stenting.

(A6) TNM staging; MDT outcome and patient preference.

Colorectal surgery

Case I

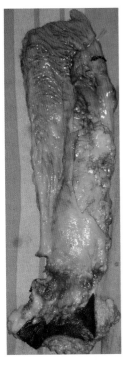

Figure 3.1a

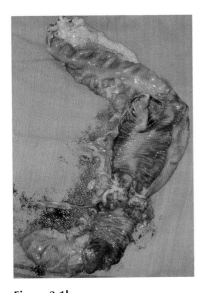

Figure 3.1b

Questions

Q1 Identify and describe the surgical specimen shown in Figure 3.1a.

Q2 Identify and describe the surgical specimen shown in Figure 3.1b.

Q3 Describe the presenting symptoms of this disease.

Q4 Is there any difference in the presentation of right-sided versus left-sided lesions?

Q5 How do you investigate and stage the disease?

Q6 Describe the staging system for this condition.

Q7 What is the five-year survival rate for this disease?

Q8 Describe the modes of spread.

Q9 Describe the treatment options available.

Q10 What are the prognostic factors of colorectal cancers?

Q11 What do you understand by the term TME?

Q12 Is there a role for local therapy alone for rectal cancer?

Answers

(A1) This is a surgical specimen of an abdomino-perineal excision of rectum (APER) for a low rectal cancer, containing part of sigmoid colon, entire rectum with the tumour, and anal canal.

(A2) This is a surgical specimen of descending colon containing an obstructing tumour with proximal dilatation.

(A3) Can present with either chronic symptoms or as an emergency.
- Chronic symptoms: change in bowel habit in the form of alternating constipation and diarrhoea, bleeding per rectum (PR), tenesmus and iron deficiency anaemia.
- Emergency: intestinal obstruction, overt rectal bleeding and colonic perforation either at the site of the tumour or at caecum secondary to closed loop obstruction.

(A4) Yes.
- Right-sided colonic tumours usually present late as the tumour can reach large size without causing pain or appreciable change in bowel habit owing to the capacious and distensible nature of the right colon and the fluid consistency of the stools. Commonly patients with right-sided tumours present with symptoms of iron deficiency anaemia.
- Left-sided colonic tumours usually present early, in the form of appreciable change in bowel habit or as bowel obstruction owing to the less distensible nature of the left colon and the solid consistency of the stool.
- Typically rectal cancer can present as bleeding per rectum, tenesmus sensation of incomplete defaecation or change in bowel habit. It can also present with rectal pain in locally advanced cases.

(A5) To confirm the diagnosis:
- clinical examination in the form of digital rectal examination (DRE) and abdominal examination: DRE can identify tumours in the lower rectum, and abdominal examination may at times reveal a palpable tumour mass
- proctosigmoidoscopy: can be performed in the outpatient clinic, can identify tumours in the rectum and can aid in taking biopsies
- colonoscopy: can reach up to caecum and is helpful in identifying the probable site of lesion, taking biopsies and identifying synchronous lesions
- barium enema: able to identify lesions up to caecum but unable to take biopsies
- CT colonography: able to identify lesions up to caecum but unable to take biopsies. Also able to stage the disease.

To stage the disease:
- CT scan of chest, abdomen and pelvis: identify lung metastasis, malignant pleural effusions, liver metastasis, ascites and local extrarectal spread in case of rectal cancers as well as adjoining organ involvement in the form of anterior abdominal wall infiltration, uterus, bladder, seminal vesicles, infiltration into pancreas, etc.
- MRI scan of pelvis and perineum: mandatory in cases of rectal tumours. Able to

assess mesorectal involvement, mesorectal lymphadenopathy and pelvic side wall
involvement
- transrectal ultrasound scan: to assess the depth of tumour penetration (T stage) in
  case of rectal cancers
- radionuclide bone scan: necessary if suspicion of bony metastasis arises
- MRI/PET scan of liver: necessary if liver lesions are doubtful and non-confirmatory on
  CT scan.

(A6) Dukes staging – commonly used staging system to prognosticate and for treatment
planning:
- Stage A – tumour confined to the bowel wall (including the muscularis propria)
- Stage B – tumour penetrating the muscularis propria with no involvement of lymph
  nodes
- Stage C1 – only regional lymph nodes involved
- Stage C2 – lymph node at the point of ligature involved by tumour.

Other staging systems are the TNM and Astler–Coller classification.

(A7) Five-year survival rate in resected colorectal cancer with curative intent is:
Duke's A – 90%
Duke's B – 60%
Duke's C – 40%
Severe dysplasia/intramucosal carcinoma is close to 100%.

(A8) The various modes of spread are:
- *direct local spread*: intramural spread or involvement of adjacent organs, e.g.
  duodenum, stomach, spleen, pelvic organs
- *lymphatic spread*: most common spread – follows the pathway of blood vessels
- *haematogenous spread*: spread to liver, lungs
- *transcoelomic spread*: via body cavities, i.e. transperitoneal – rare but can happen
  and associated with grave prognosis.

(A9) The various treatment options available are surgery, radiotherapy, and chemotherapy.
- Surgical options include removal of the colon containing the tumour, based on the
  vascular supply. Example:
  - right hemicolectomy for right-sided cancers, left hemicolectomy for left-sided
    cancers and extended right hemicolectomy for cancers involving hepatic flexure
    and transverse colon
  - sigmoid colectomy for sigmoid cancers
  - for rectal cancers, commonly performed surgical procedures are anterior
    resection which can be low or ultra-low based on the tumour location and
    abdomino-perineal excision of rectum (APER) for low rectal cancers where safe
    surgical margins cannot be given or if sphincter is involved or preservation is not
    possible.
- Radiotherapy is mainly offered in rectal cancers, either preoperative or postoperative
  depending upon the local staging of the tumour and postoperative margins.

- Chemotherapy is offered for all node-positive colorectal tumours postoperatively, and for selected cases of rectal cancer it is offered preoperatively along with radiotherapy.

(A10) Staging – TNM/Dukes.
Tumour differentiation.
Lymphovascular invasion.
Adequacy of resection in case of rectal cancers.

(A11) Total mesorectal excision.
Described by Sir Bill Heald in 1979, this concept emphasises full mesorectal clearance. The retrorectal space is entered between the mesorectum and the presacral fascia and sharp dissection is continued to about 3 or 4 cm below the lower border of the growth. The sharp technique used ensures that the specimen contains intact mesorectum with negative tumour margins in the majority of resectable rectal cancers. The technique allows the preservation of pelvic autonomic nerves, reducing sexual and urinary dysfunction. It has been suggested that this technique reduces local recurrence rates.

(A12) Yes.
The earliest procedures done on rectal tumours were local. Endoscopic Rectal Ultrasound (ERUS) and MRI pelvis has renewed interest in local therapy for these cancers. Patient selection is the most important factor. The following factors should be taken into consideration:
- tumours ≤4 cm
- fixed tumours are not appropriate. Fixation indicates the tumour has penetrated the wall
- selected cases of T1 lesions only. Mesorectal nodal involvement is as high as 66% for T3 tumours and therefore local treatment is not an option
- tumours with proven mesorectal nodes are not appropriate for local resection
- local control and survival appear to be worse in patients with lymphovascular and perineural invasion.

Digital rectal examination, proctoscopy and biopsy of the lesion along with ERUS help to evaluate the depth of invasion of the rectal wall (T stage) and nodal status.

Local procedures commonly done are:
- full thickness excision
  - posterior approaches
    transsacral resection – Kraske procedure
    transsphincteric resection – York–Mason procedure
  - transanal approaches
    transanal excision
    transanal endoscopic microsurgery (TEM)
- ablative procedures such as electrocoagulation and endocavity radiation have been used as local therapy.

Case 2

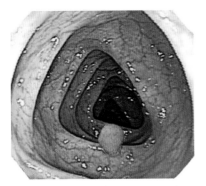

Figure 3.2a

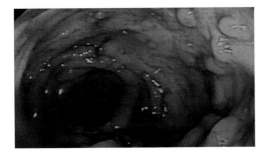

Figure 3.2b

Questions

Q1 Describe what you see in Figure 3.2a and Figure 3.2b, both taken at colonoscopy.

Q2 How do you classify this problem?

Q3 Explain the salient features of each type.

Q4 How can they present?

Q5 How would you manage this problem?

Q6 What do you understand about the adenoma–carcinoma sequence?

Answers

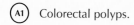 Colorectal polyps.

A2 Colorectal polyps can be broadly classified as:
- inflammatory
- hamartomatous
- metaplastic
- adenomatous.

A3 a) *Inflammatory polyps*:
- form from an island of hypertrophied mucosa in an area of inflammation and ulceration
- they are sometimes referred as pseudopolyps
- occur in ulcerative colitis, Crohn's colitis, diverticulitis, chronic dysentery and benign lymphomatous lesions of the colon.

b) *Hamartomatous polyps* are found in two forms:
- juvenile polyps are found in infants and children, often multiple and pedunculated, familial and majority of them occur in rectum and distal sigmoid colon
- Peutz–Jeghers syndrome is associated with pigmented lesions on the face and on the buccal and lingual mucosa. It is a familial condition and the polyps are always multiple, found more commonly in the small bowel, and have a significant malignant potential.

c) *Metaplastic (hyperplastic) polyps*:
- plaque-like growths which rarely exceed 5 mm
- most commonly found in the rectum
- rarely symptomatic and not premalignant.

d) *Adenomatous polyps*:
- benign neoplastic growths arising from the mucosa of the intestine
- can occur anywhere in the GI tract, but most commonly in rectum and left colon
- further classified into tubular, villous and tubulo-villous adenomas
- in general villous adenomas are more likely to undergo malignant change.

These polyps could be sessile or pedunculated.

A4 Asymptomatic.
Rectal bleeding.
Mucous discharge PR.
Spurious diarrhoea.
Malignant change and clinical features of CRC (*see* Case 1).

A5 Endoscopic polypectomy is the mainstay of treatment. For flat adenomas low in the rectum, TEMS (Transanal Endoscopic Micro Surgery) could be attempted. All the resected polyps should be carefully assessed histologically for evidence of malignant change. Following benign polyp removal, based on the size and number, patients should be kept under colonoscopic surveillance.

 Adenoma–carcinoma sequence is associated with an orderly progression of genetic mutations allowing transformation of normal colonic mucosa to carcinoma. The mutations involve APC gene (Adenomatous Polyposis Coli), K-ras gene, DCC gene (deleted in colorectal cancer) and p53 tumour suppressor gene.

Your revision notes

Case 3

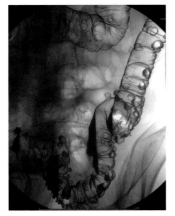

Figure 3.3a

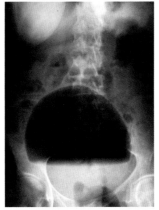

Figure 3.3b

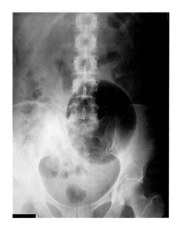

Figure 3.3c

Questions

Q1 What investigation has been performed in Figure 3.3a and what does it demonstrate?

Q2 What is meant by a diverticulum?

Q3 How do you classify them? Give examples.

Q4 What is the aetiology of colonic diverticulosis?

Q5 What are the clinical features of sigmoid diverticular disease? What does Figure 3.3b show? What has happened?

Q6 What investigative modalities are available for diverticulosis?

Q7 How would you manage sigmoid diverticular disease?

Q8 What radiographic sign is being demonstrated in Figure 3.3c and what does it signify?

Answers

(A1) The investigation shown is a double contrast barium enema and it shows multiple colonic diverticula.

(A2) A diverticulum is an abnormal outpouching of a hollow viscus into the surrounding tissues.

(A3) Can be classified as true or false diverticulum.
- True – contains all layers of the bowel wall.
  - Origin: congenital
  - Example: Meckel's diverticulum
- False – does not contain all layers of bowel wall.
  - Origin: acquired
  - Example: colonic diverticulum

(A4) Colonic diverticulosis is an acquired diverticular disease caused by increased intraluminal pressure leading to outpouching of colonic mucosa. This characteristically occurs at sites of weakness where mesenteric blood vessels pass between the muscle of the taenia coli.

Incidence: 30% chance at 60 years of age, 60% chance at 80 years and older.

Distribution: sigmoid colon (45%); sigmoid and descending colon (35%); 10% affecting sigmoid, descending and transverse; 5% pan colonic; caecum (5%).

Causes: lack of adequate dietary fibre (thereby decreasing the stool weight and causing hard consistency) leads to increased segmentation pressure in the sigmoid colon which causes mucosal outpouching resulting in diverticulum.

(A5) Asymptomatic (symptoms occur only when the diverticulum is inflamed)
Acute presentation:
- acute diverticulitis
- diverticular abscess
- diverticular bleedings manifesting as bleeding PR
- diverticular perforation presenting as peritonitis
- large bowel obstruction secondary to diverticular stricture.

Chronic presentation:
- chronic lower abdominal pain
- involvement of adjacent organs forming a mass (which can present at times as acute phlegmon) or forming fistula with small bowel, bladder (Figure 3.3b), uterus, vagina
- malignant change.

Figure 3.3b – pneumaturia – likely colovesical fistula as a complication of diverticular disease.

Colonoscopy/flexible sigmoidoscopy.
Barium enema.
CT scan of abdomen and pelvis/CT pneumocolon.

Colonoscopy/flexible sigmoidoscopy and barium enema is performed in non-acute situations as the risk of perforation of an inflamed diverticulum is higher. But in bleeding PR, colonoscopy can be performed with caution.

CT scan is performed in acute situations – can reveal inflamed diverticulum, associated diverticular abscess and any evidence of perforation. Also useful to evaluate complicated diverticular disease like diverticular mass, adjacent organ involvement and fistulating disease.

- Asymptomatic sigmoid diverticular disease can be managed conservatively with high-fibre diet.
- Acute sigmoid diverticulitis can be conservatively managed initially with IV antibiotics. If it fails to improve, CT scan has to be performed to identify complications like diverticular abscess, then managed accordingly.
- Diverticular abscess, if localised, can be managed by image-guided drainage, and elective sigmoid resection can be performed later.
- Sigmoid diverticular perforation with resultant purulent or faecal peritonitis can be safely managed by emergency sigmoid resection and Hartmann's procedure.
- Sigmoid diverticular bleeding can be managed conservatively initially. If the bleeding leads to haemodynamic instability, the situation generally leads to sigmoid resection.
- In cases of adjacent organ involvement, after adequate investigation, elective sigmoid resection has to be performed.
- For chronic indolent cases with recurrent episodes of acute diverticulitis that resolve with antibiotic therapy, after three or more such episodes in a year, elective sigmoid resection has to be considered as the incidence of complication in such groups is significantly higher.

 Figure 3.3c – The 'balloon sign' (air-filled cyst).
Indicates there is an underlying giant colonic diverticulum. This is a rare complication of diverticular disease of the colon and is thought to result from a 'ball-valve effect'. Most common symptoms are abdominal pain, a palpable abdominal mass, and many patients present acutely with complications such as perforation and peritonitis. Preoperative diagnosis requires a high degree of suspicion and needs to be differentiated from a sigmoid volvulus, caecal volvulus and intestinal duplication cyst. There is a high incidence of complications and treatment is advised even in asymptomatic cases – consists of excision of the cyst with resection of the adjacent colon with primary anastomosis (sigmoid colectomy).

Your revision notes

Case 4

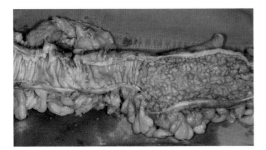

Figure 3.4a

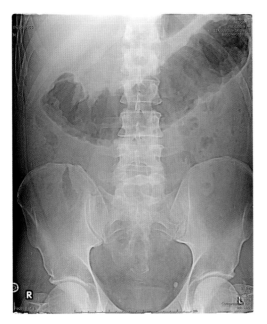

Figure 3.4b

Questions

Q1 Describe what Figure 3.4a shows. Figure 3.4b is an X-ray taken from the same patient preoperatively. What does it show?

Q2 What's the most likely diagnosis?

Q3 What are the typical microscopic appearances of this disease?

Q4 What are the typical clinical features of this condition?

Q5 What are the extra-intestinal manifestations of this condition?

Q6 What are the main complications of this disease?

Q7 How is this condition treated?

Q8 What are the indications for surgery in this condition?

Q9 What biochemical markers are indicative of a severe episode and what clinical features suggest a poor prognosis?

Q10 What surgical options are available for the elective management of this condition?

Answers

(A1) On gross examination this macroscopic specimen consists of an opened colon, showing ulceration including prominent cobblestone ulceration, which is more extensive on one side. The other edge of the specimen has normal mucosa with minimal cobblestoning and ulceration The wall is thickened and shows some discolouration, possibly as the result of a perforation. Ulceration is evident between cobblestoning as well as in the adjacent area.

AXR: dilated transverse colon with mucosal oedema, featureless appearance, lack of haustra, signs of toxic megacolon.

(A2) Ulcerative colitis.

(A3) Acute and chronic inflammatory infiltrate, formation of crypt abscesses and eventual distortion of crypt lining.

(A4) Commonest presentation is bloody diarrhoea with marked faecal urgency. This may be associated with abdominal pain (although pain is more often a feature of Crohn's disease), malaise, anorexia and weight loss.

(A5) Related to the intestinal disease activity:
- pyoderma gangrenosum
- erythema nodosum
- aphthous ulcers of the mouth and vagina
- iritis
- large joint arthritis.

Unrelated to the intestinal disease activity:
- sacroiliitis
- ankylosing spondylitis
- chronic active hepatitis
- cirrhosis
- sclerosing cholangitis
- cholangiocarcinoma
- fingernail clubbing.

(A6) Massive haemorrhage.
Toxic megacolon.
Colonic perforation.
Colonic stricture.
Perianal suppuration.
Giant inflammatory polyposis syndrome.
Colonic carcinoma.

(A7) Treatment is primarily medical:
- acute attacks – use of steroids to induce remission, which is then maintained by 5-aminosalicyclic acid (5-ASA) derivatives such as mesalazine
- localised proctitis may be treated with foam enemas of either steroids or 5-ASA
- widespread disease requires oral or IV therapy. Treatments such as oral budesonide and azathioprine have been used to reduce the impact of steroid therapy. Important also to improve nutrition levels using enteral and parenteral means.

(A8) Surgical indications:
- refractory to medical therapy. Signified by recurrent attacks, rapidly relapsing disease on maximal medical therapy or where the disease is causing chronic disability or failure to thrive
- steroid-dependent or steroid-resistant cases
- if a severe attack of colitis does not respond within 48 hours of maximal medical therapy then an urgent colectomy must be considered. Factors to be considered include eight or more bloody stool motions per day, persistent tachycardia, fever above 38.5°, dilatation of the colon more than 5 cm or increasing diameter on serial films, and a falling albumin
- acute complications of the disease – toxic dilatation, perforation or uncontrollable haemorrhage (rare)
- prophylaxis – UC increases the risk of colonic adenocarcinoma. The risk is thought to be 1% at 10 years, 5% at 20 years and 10% at 25 years of disease
- presence of dysplasia in colonoscopic biopsy is an indication for colectomy.

(A9) High CRP and ESR and low haemoglobin and albumin signifying severe inflammation. Poor prognostic features include severe initial attack, late-onset disease and disease affecting the whole of the colon.

(A10) Elective surgery options:
- panproctocolectomy and ileostomy: advantage of a single operation and no surveillance required. Disadvantages are longer operation associated with higher complications and permanent end stoma especially in young patients
- subtotal colectomy and ileorectal anastomosis (if rectal sparing): advantage of a single procedure and no stoma. However, results in residual rectum with possibility of recurrent disease and cancer risk requiring surveillance. Appropriate if rectum is only mildly affected
- panproctocolectomy and ileal anal pouch reconstruction: usually patient is continent and all diseased segment is removed. Often more than one operation required and complications are common (30%) in the form of pouchitis.

Hence each option has to be tailored to the individual patient.

Your revision notes

Case 5

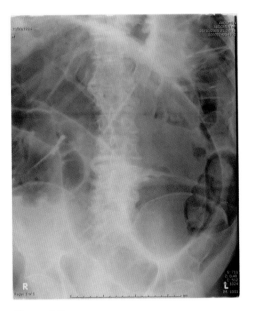

Figure 3.5a

Questions

Q1 Look at Figure 3.5a. This elderly patient presented with abdominal distension and complete obstruction. What does this X-ray show?

Q2 What are the risk factors for developing this condition?

Q3 What further investigations may help?

Q4 What are the complications of this condition?

Q5 How would you manage this condition? What has happened in Figure 3.5b in a different patient?

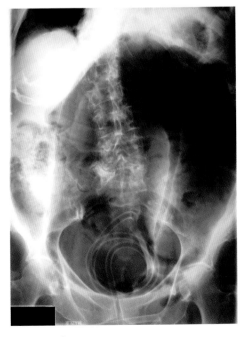

Figure 3.5b

Answers

(A1) Massively distended large bowel with 'coffee bean' shaped appearance consistent with sigmoid volvulus.

(A2) Elderly males who are typically hospitalised with previous history of chronic constipation, laxative abuse and unrelated medical problems. Predisposing factors include a long sigmoid loop with a narrow mesentery. In addition, chronic constipation, a high-fibre diet and systemic neurological disease are important.

(A3) Gastrografin (water-soluble) enema – can see a 'bird–beak' narrowing at the point of obstruction.

(A4) Massive abdominal distension with respiratory embarrassment.
Gangrene and perforation.
Faecal peritonitis.

(A5) a) *Acute*:
- relatively fit and healthy individuals: sigmoid resection and Hartmann's procedure or primary anastomosis in both acute situations and chronic recurrent cases
- relatively unfit, elderly, demented patients with multiple co-morbidities: initially, decompression can be gently and very carefully attempted with flatus tube or flexible sigmoidoscopy with minimal air insufflation.

b) *Chronic cases*:
- relatively fit and healthy individuals can be better served by sigmoid resection and Hartmann's procedure or primary anastomosis
- for recurrent cases, percutaneous endoscopic sigmoidopexy (PES) should be considered.

Figure 3.5b: Sigmoid volvulus with placement of a rectal tube.

Case 6

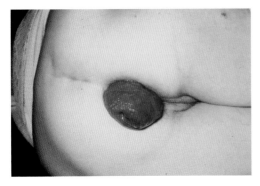

Figure 3.6

Questions

Q1 What is the diagnosis in this 75-year-old woman?

Q2 How do you classify this condition and how do you differentiate between the subtypes?

Q3 What are the aetiological and predisposing factors?

Q4 What are the usual symptoms that patients with this condition experience?

Q5 What are the complications of this condition?

Q6 Does this condition need any investigations prior to management?

Q7 How would you manage this condition?

Answers

(A1) Full-thickness rectal prolapse.

(A2) Rectal prolapse can be classified as full-thickness or complete rectal prolapse, and partial-thickness or incomplete rectal prolapse. Full-thickness prolapse involves prolapse of the entire thickness of the rectal wall whereas partial-thickness rectal prolapse involves prolapse of only the mucosa of the rectal wall.

Both conditions can be differentiated by the finger test. On digital examination using the index finger and thumb, full-thickness rectal prolapse feels like a double-layered tube.

(A3) Partial-thickness rectal prolapse occurs due to laxity of the tissue in the rectal submucosa leading to abnormal mobility of the rectal mucosa on the underlying circular muscle. Full-thickness rectal prolapse occurs due to laxity of the pelvic floor musculature.

Predisposing factors in children include poor toilet training, chronic constipation or chronic diarrhoea and malnutrition. Predisposing factors in adults include conditions causing weak pelvic floor musculature, e.g. multiparous women, obstetric trauma, somatic denervation of the sphincter and pelvic floor muscle due to neuropathy.

(A4) Lump that prolapses on defaecation, which either reduces spontaneously or requires manual reduction.
Perianal discomfort.
Mucus discharge per rectum.
Faecal incontinence.
PR bleeding.

(A5) Strangulation as a result of incarceration due to difficulty in reduction. Acute urinary retention.

(A6) Yes.
- Elderly patients presenting with this condition need flexible sigmoidoscopy to rule out a proximal malignancy.
- Young female patients presenting with this condition along with features of obstructed defaecation need defaecating proctogram to assess the severity of prolapse and the presence of associated enterocoele, which will help in planning appropriate surgical intervention.
- In very young patients, endoanal ultrasound with pudendal nerve latency assessment has to be performed to identify any associated anatomical and neurological abnormality that could have a significant impact on the outcome of any planned surgical intervention.

Management is usually surgical in fit patients. Surgical approach can be broadly classified into abdominal and perineal procedures.
- Abdominal procedures: can be performed in fit and healthy individuals:
    - abdominal rectopexy – suture or mesh – open or laparoscopic
    - resection rectopexy – resection of redundant sigmoid colon followed by fixation of rectum with either sutures or mesh.

Recurrence rates are very low compared to perineal procedures but have to be balanced against the risks of general anaesthesia and the morbidity of rectal mobilisation, especially in male patients – the chances of sexual and bladder dysfunction.
- Perineal procedures: can be performed in elderly, frail patients:
    - perineal rectosigmoidectomy – with placation of levator ani (Altemeier's procedure)
    - Delorme's procedure – plication procedure
    - stapled transanal rectal resection (STARR).

Recurrence rates are slightly higher than the abdominal procedures but have to be balanced by the fact that these procedures can be performed in regional anaesthesia with less postoperative morbidity.

Your revision notes

Case 7

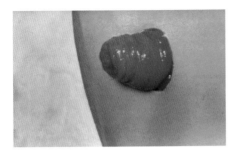

Figure 3.7a

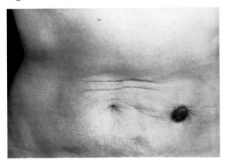

Figure 3.7b

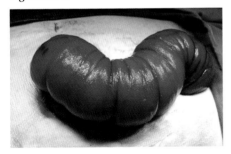

Figure 3.7c

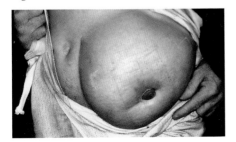

Figure 3.7d

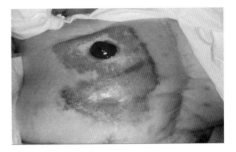

Figure 3.7e

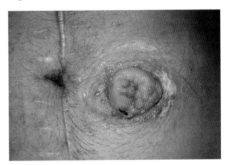

Figure 3.7f

Questions

Q1 Figures 3.7a and 3.7b depict two different types of stoma. What are they called?

Q2 What are the indications for forming a stoma?

Q3 What factors determine stoma location?

Q4 What are the differences between an ileostomy and a colostomy?

Q5 Figures 3.7c, 3.7d, 3.7e and 3.7f show possible complications of a stoma. What are they?

Answers

(A1) Figure 3.7a – End ileostomy.
Figure 3.7b – End colostomy.

(A2) Diversion:
- defunction a distal anastomosis
  - previously contaminated bowel
  - technical considerations – low anterior resection or ileorectal anastomosis
- urinary diversion following cystectomy.

Exteriorisation:
- perforated or contaminated bowel, e.g. distal abscesses/fistula
- permanent stoma, e.g. APER.

Feeding, e.g. percutaneous endoscopic gastrostomy (PEG).
Lavage: appendicostomy for large bowel washout.
Decompression.

(A3) Stoma site:
- 5 cm from umbilicus
- away from scars or skin creases
- away from bony prominences or waistline of clothes
- site that is easy for patient to access – not under a large fold of fat!
- stoma must be within the rectus abdominis
- need to consider patient's mobility and eyesight.

(A4) Ileostomy versus colostomy

Characteristic	Ileostomy	Colostomy
Typical site	RIF	LIF
Surface	Spout	Flush with skin
Contents	Watery – small bowel	Faeculent
Effluent	Continuous	Intermittent
Permanent	Panproctocolectomy	APER
Temporary	Loop ileostomy after low anterior resection	Hartmann's procedure

(A5) Figure 3.7c – stomal prolapse.
Figure 3.7d – parastomal hernia.
Figure 3.7e – peristomal skin excoriation.
Figure 3.7f – stomal carcinoma.

Specific complications:
- ischaemia and gangrene
- haemorrhage
- retraction
- prolapse/intussusception

- parastomal hernia
- stenosis – leads to constipation
- peristomal skin excoriation
- stomal cancer.

General complications– related to underlying disease:
- stoma diarrhoea – water and electrolyte imbalance, hypokalaemia
- nutritional disorders
- stones – both gallstones and renal stones more common after ileostomy
- psychosexual
- residual disease, e.g. Crohn's and parastomal fistula, metastasis.

Your revision notes

Case 8

A 65-year-old lady presented to A&E with a four-day history of diarrhoea following antibiotic treatment for a chest infection two weeks prior. She underwent a rigid sigmoidoscopy (Figure 3.8a) as part of her initial assessment. Figure 3.8b shows the colectomy specimen taken when she failed to respond to conservative treatment and developed signs of toxic megacolon.

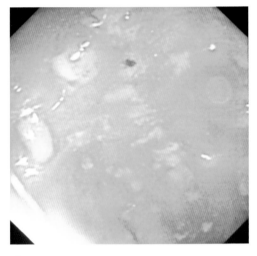

Figure 3.8a

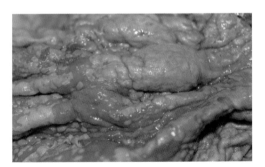

Figure 3.8b

Questions

Q1 Describe what you see on the rigid sigmoidoscopy examination (Figure 3.8a) and on the colonic specimen (Figure 3.8b). What is the clinical condition?

Q2 What are the clinical features of this condition?

Q3 What are the underlying risk factors for developing this type of diarrhoea?

Q4 What factors are highly suggestive of the diagnosis?

Q5 What are the principles of management?

Answers

(A1) Rigid sigmoidoscopy shows yellow patches on the rectal/colonic mucosa typical of pseudomembranes.

The specimen reveals multiple exudative punctate raised yellow plaques with intervening areas of oedematous mucosa.

The clinical condition is pseudomembranous enterocolitis.

(A2) Pseudomembranous enterocolitis is caused by a gram-positive anaerobic bacillus *Clostridium difficile* following antibiotic usage. It is associated with almost all antibiotics, although ampicillin, amoxicillin, clindamycin and lincomycin account for the majority of cases. *Clostridium difficile* can cause a less severe infection manifesting as self-limiting diarrhoea, and a more severe infection in the form of pseudomembranous colitis manifesting as severe bloody diarrhoea associated with marked abdominal pain, fever and tenesmus. Extreme cases can present as abdominal distension secondary to toxic dilatation of the colon and peritonitis secondary to colonic perforation.

(A3) History of antibiotic use in the last 10 weeks especially use of ampicillin, clindamycin, and cephalosporins (especially third-generation – cefotaxime, ceftriaxone and ceftazidime).

Risk is less with other antibiotics but all antibiotics, including metronidazole and vancomycin, have been associated with *C. difficile*-associated diarrhoea (CDAD).

Antineoplastic agents.

Age >60 years.

Gastrointestinal surgery.

Enemas, stool softeners.

Enteral feeding – especially postpyloric.

(A4) Elevated white cell count (WCC) is common (50–60%) and can be marked (WCC >30 000/mm³).

Elevation of WCC may precede the onset of the diarrhoea or abdominal discomfort.

Low serum albumin levels from protein-losing enteropathy is common and has been associated with a poor prognosis.

Specific diagnosis is made with enzyme immunoassay (EIA) to detect toxin A and B

There is no indication for serial monitoring of stools or end-of-treatment test of cure for *C. difficile* toxin.

(A5) Management principles:
- isolation of the patient
- fluid and electrolyte balance
- discontinue the antibiotic suspected to have been responsible
- if antibiotics cannot be discontinued change to antibiotic with less propensity to cause CDAD, e.g. aminoglycosides, quinolones or macrolides
- if CDAD mild – observation without specific treatment is reasonable – relapse has not been noted after spontaneous resolution (20–25% cases)

- avoid antimotility drugs – can worsen disease and give false sense of response to therapy
- oral metronidazole for 10–14 days is the initial drug of choice (cure rate 95%, recurrence 5–15%)
- oral vancomycin (125 mg qds) should be substituted if no improvement in three to five days (recommended first line in pregnancy and lactation)
- patients who cannot tolerate oral agents – IV metronidazole drug of choice
- vancomycin via retention enema can be used
- no indication for treatment of patients with asymptomatic carrier state
- surgical intervention (colectomy) for severe, resistant cases.

Your revision notes

Case 9

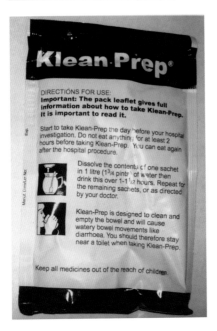

Figure 3.9a

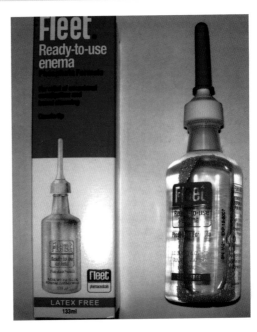

Figure 3.9c

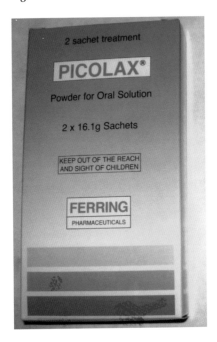

Figure 3.9b

Questions

(Q1) What do the pictures show and for what purpose(s) are they used?

(Q2) What is meant by bowel preparation and how is it given?

(Q3) What are the commonly used bowel preparation agents and how do they act?

(Q4) What are the indications for bowel preparation?

(Q5) What are the complications of bowel preparation, if any?

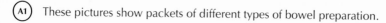

Answers

(A1) These pictures show packets of different types of bowel preparation.

(A2) Bowel preparation usually signifies cleansing of large bowel prior to a procedure. It can be done by oral administration of agents that act on the large bowel or by rectal administration of agents that act as stimulants.

(A3) The commonly used bowel preparation agents are polyethylene glycol, sodium picosulphate, and magnesium sulphate.
- Polyethylene glycol acts by osmotic activity, which promotes colonic mucosal secretion of fluid, producing diarrhoea.
- Sodium picosulphate and magnesium sulphate act as stimulant laxatives.
- Phosphate enema acts as a stimulant laxative.

(A4) Bowel preparation is usually performed for left-sided colonic procedures like left hemicolectomy, sigmoid resection, anterior resection of rectum and transanal endoscopic microsurgery (TEMS) with the exception of APER.

Right-sided colonic procedures do not require bowel preparation.

Oesophageal resection with colonic interposition (coloplasty) also requires bowel preparation.

Usually bowel preparation is done preoperatively and in some cases, especially in emergency situations, can be performed intraoperatively.

Colonic investigations like colonoscopy, barium enema and CT colonography require bowel preparation. Flexible sigmoidoscopy requires only a phosphate enema one to two hours prior to the procedure.

Traditionally, bowel preparation is used with a view to reducing the rates of anastomotic dehiscence, and for aesthetic reasons (when handling the bowel intraoperatively). But recent randomised studies have challenged the traditional belief and have shown that bowel preparation may not be necessary even for left-sided colonic procedures and have also shown that bowel preparation delays postoperative recovery.

(A5) Complications of bowel preparation include electrolyte disturbances but the current bowel preparation agents come with electrolyte supplements that minimise this problem.

Case 10

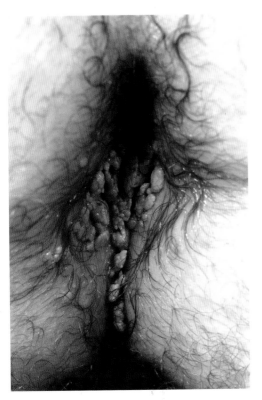

Figure 3.10

Questions

Q1 Look at Figure 3.10. What is the differential diagnosis? What is the most likely diagnosis?

Q2 What is the causative agent? What is the significance of this?

Q3 Which group of people is most affected by this problem?

Q4 What does the patient complain of?

Q5 What treatments are available?

Answers

(A1) Perianal warts (condylomata acuminata) – most likely diagnosis.
Molluscum contagiosum – small, raised, centrally umbilicated, pinkish-white lesions caused by a pox virus.
Condylomata latum (secondary syphilitic sores).
Hypertrophied anal papillae.

(A2) Human papillomavirus (HPV) Types 6, 11, 16 and 18.
Potential premalignant type of HPV. Subtypes 16 and 18 behave more aggressively and have been more frequently associated with dysplasia and malignant transformation.

(A3) Homosexual males. This condition is invariably sexually transmitted.

(A4) Perianal lumps, itching, bleeding, anal discharge, persistent perianal wetness and pain.

(A5) Cryotherapy.
Immunotherapy – intralesional injection of d-interferon.
Surgical excision.
All treatment options are associated with high recurrence rates (10–75%).

Case 11

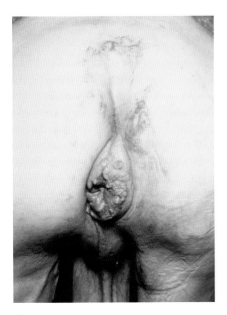

Figure 3.11a

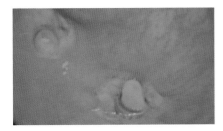

Figure 3.11b

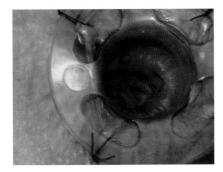

Figure 3.11c

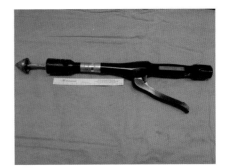

Figure 3.11d

Questions

- **Q1** Identify the perianal condition in Figure 3.11a.
- **Q2** Define this condition.
- **Q3** How do you classify this condition?
- **Q4** What are the clinical features of this problem?
- **Q5** What are the complications?
- **Q6** How do you investigate this condition?
- **Q7** How do you manage this condition non-operatively? What has happened in Figure 3.11b?
- **Q8** What are the operative options? What procedure is depicted in Figures 3.11c and 3.11d? Does it have any advantages?
- **Q9** What are the possible postoperative complications of conventional surgery?

Answers

(A1) The perianal condition is thrombosed, prolapsed haemorrhoids.

(A2) Haemorrhoids are prolapsed anal cushions in the anal canal resulting from degeneration of the smooth muscle and fibro-elastic tissues that support the anal cushions. The aetiology for the degeneration is not precisely known but chronic constipation and straining are recognised contributing factors.

(A3) Haemorrhoids can be classified clinically as follows:
1st degree: internal haemorrhoids, which can be visualised only on proctoscopic examination, presenting with bleeding alone
2nd degree: haemorrhoids that prolapse on defaecation but reduce spontaneously
3rd degree: haemorrhoids that prolapse and require manual reduction
4th degree: irreducibly prolapsed haemorrhoids.

(A4) The most common symptom is painless, bright red rectal bleeding following immediately after defaecation. Haemorrhoids can also present with pruritus, perianal swelling and minor soiling. Pain from haemorrhoids is associated with complications.

(A5) The complications of haemorrhoids are:
• thrombosis leading to severe pain
• massive haemorrhage
• minor incontinence due to poor sealing owing to displaced anal cushions.

(A6) Perianal examination can reveal 3rd and 4th degree haemorrhoids. Digital rectal examination will usually be normal. Proctoscopy can reveal the presence or absence, as well as the extent of involvement, of haemorrhoids. In selected cases, when there is any doubt about the source of bleeding, flexible sigmoidoscopy/barium enema/colonoscopy should be performed to exclude a proximal source.

(A7) Asymptomatic haemorrhoids do not need any intervention apart from reassurance after excluding serious disease.

Symptomatic haemorrhoids can be treated by various non-operative, outpatient procedures as well as operative procedures. The most common outpatient, non-operative procedures include injection sclerotherapy, rubber band ligation (Figure 3.11b). Other techniques include infrared photocoagulation, laser photocoagulation, bipolar coagulation and cryotherapy.

(A8) Operative procedures include open/closed haemorrhoidectomy (Milligan–Morgan/ Ferguson). The underlying principle of the Milligan–Morgan haemorrhoidectomy is the preservation of skin bridges between the excised haemorrhoids to prevent stricturing. Regardless of the method of excision, the resultant wounds are left to heal by secondary intention (open haemorrhoidectomy). In the closed haemorrhoidectomy, first described by Ferguson and Heaton in 1959, the haemorrhoidal plexus is dissected from the internal sphincter, and the wounds closed primarily with an absorbable suture. With either the

Milligan–Morgan or the Ferguson technique, there is inevitably an anocutaneous wound, which is associated with postoperative pain, morbidity and impairment of function.

Figures 3.11c and 3.11d (stapler) demonstrate the stapled haemorrhoidopexy technique. It was the first attempt to deal with the problem of haemorrhoidal prolapse by re-suspending the prolapsed tissue and avoiding an anocutaneous wound. The stapling device, developed in the 1990s, shortens the prolapsing mucosa (and thus reduces the haemorrhoids) and interrupts branches of the haemorrhoidal vessels.

Stapled haemorrhoidopexy reduces the length of hospital stay and may have an advantage in terms of decreased operating time, reduced postoperative pain and less bleeding but is associated with an increased rate of recurrent prolapse. The avoidance of an anocutaneous wound might contribute to the reduced postoperative pain and earlier return to normal activities reported in some randomised trials. However, there is limited long-term data available, and therefore, the durability of stapled haemorrhoidopexy remains unclear.

Another procedure is HALO (Haemorrhoidal Arterial Ligation Operation) under Doppler guidance.

Thrombosed prolapsed haemorrhoids can initially be managed conservatively, followed by operative intervention. Conservative measures include analgesics, local anaesthetic gel application, cold ice packs, bed rest and elevation of the foot of the bed. Generally an operative procedure should be avoided acutely due to potential higher postoperative complications such as sepsis.

 The complications of haemorrhoidectomy are:
- pain
- bleeding
- acute urinary retention
- perianal sepsis
- anal stricture.

Your revision notes

Case 12

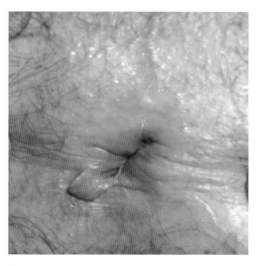

Figure 3.12

Questions

(Q1) What condition is shown in
Figure 3.12?

(Q2) What is the definition of this
condition and how does it develop?

(Q3) What are the clinical features?

(Q4) How do you make a diagnosis?

(Q5) How do you manage this problem?

Answers

 Anal fissure.

 An anal fissure is a linear ulcer which occurs in the anal canal just distal to the dentate line. Most commonly it's a primary condition but it can also be caused by Crohn's disease, trauma or malignancy.

The main underlying pathology is the high resting anal pressure caused by increased internal sphincter tone. As the blood supply of the anal canal passes through the internal sphincter, spasm of this muscle reduces the blood flow and oxygen tension in the skin of the anal canal leading to ischaemia. The initiating factor could be minor anal trauma caused by passage of constipated stool.

(A3) Symptoms:
- painful defaecation ('like passing glass')
- associated bright red bleeding
- pruritus ani
- mucus discharge PR.

Signs:
- perianal skin tag
- ulcer will usually be seen in the posterior midline of the anal canal
- in female patients, can be seen in the anterior midline as well.

(A4) Mainly based on the history, but confirmed by:
- perianal examination. (Digital rectal examination and proctoscopy should be avoided in a conscious patient – usually the patient will not be able to tolerate this!)
- examination under anaesthesia.

(A5) The main aim of treatment is to reduce the internal sphincter tone:
- bulk laxatives and adequate hydration
- topical application of local anaesthetics
- topical application of 0.4% glyceryl trinitrate (GTN) ointment or 2% diltiazem cream for 6–8 weeks. Response rates around 66%
- if medical treatment fails, carefully controlled lateral internal anal sphincterotomy can be done to relieve the spasm and allow healing but patient has to be warned of increased flatus and possibility of faecal incontinence.

Case 13

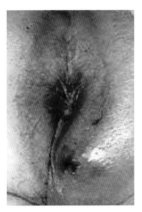

Figure 3.13a

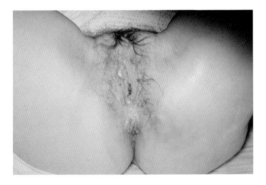

Figure 3.13b

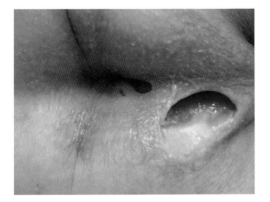

Figure 3.13c

Questions

Q1 What perianal conditions are shown in Figures 3.13a, 3.13b and 3.13c?

Q2 How do they develop?

Q3 What are the clinical features of this condition?

Q4 How would you manage this problem?

Q5 What situations require this condition to be treated promptly?

Q6 What are the complications of drainage?

Answers

(A1)   Figure 3.13a – perianal abscess.
Figure 3.13b – ischiorectal abscess.
Figure 3.13c – recurrent perianal abscess from a fistula-in-ano.

(A2)   A perianal abscess develops as a result of suppurative infection of the anal glands situated in the intersphincteric space. These glands open into the anal canal at the dentate line via a duct that traverses the internal sphincter. They get infected when the duct gets blocked and pus accumulates within the gland. The pus tracks superiorly, laterally and circumferentially, and most commonly will pass downwards in the intersphincteric plane to form a perianal abscess.

(A3)   Symptoms:
• severe perianal pain
• swelling in the perianal region
• systemic symptoms like fever and malaise.

Signs:
• tender red swelling at the anal margin
• swelling may not be evident but will be tender to touch in the perianal region.

(A4)   Management:
• analgesia
• examination under anaesthesia
• proctosigmoidoscopy to rule out an associated proctitis
• incision and drainage of the abscess taking care not to damage the sphincters. At the same time, abscess cavity should be deroofed adequately to enhance drainage. Probing and over-enthusiastic curetting should be avoided.

(A5)   Diabetic and immunocompromised patients and patients with large ischiorectal abscesses should be treated urgently to prevent the infection spreading further, leading to septicaemia and necrotising fasciitis.

(A6)   The various complications of perianal abscess drainage are:
• necrotising fasciitis
• fistula-in-ano formation (Figure 3.13c)
• transient minor incontinence of faeces and flatus.

Case 14

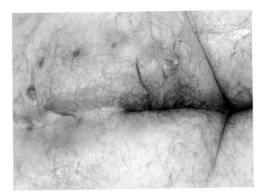

Figure 3.14

Questions

Q1 Can you identify this perianal condition?

Q2 What is the underlying pathophysiology?

Q3 How do you classify this problem?

Q4 What are the clinical features?

Q5 What is Goodsall's rule? What are the exceptions?

Q6 How do you make a diagnosis and treat this problem?

Q7 What are the specific causes of this condition?

Answers

A1 Fistula-in-ano.

A2 Fistula-in-ano is an abnormal communication between the dentate line and the perianal skin. Anal glands which are situated in the intersphincteric space open into the anal canal at the dentate line via a duct that traverses the internal sphincter. These glands get infected if the duct becomes blocked. The resulting pus accumulates within the gland and tracks superiorly, laterally and circumferentially. In the majority of cases the resulting perianal abscess discharges through the skin spontaneously or as a result of surgical intervention, and resolves. But if the duct between the gland and the dentate line becomes patent and infected, the patient will be left with a fistula-in-ano.

A3 Fistula-in-ano can be classified based on the mode of spread of anal gland infection with respect to the internal and external anal sphincter relationship.
Park's classification:
- intersphincteric
- transsphincteric
- suprasphincteric
- extrasphincteric.

A4 Symptoms:
- intermittent perianal pain
- discharge of bloodstained or purulent material
- pruritus
- recurrent episodes of pain relieved by discharge from fistula.

Signs:
- fistulous opening may be seen in the perianal region
- discharge of pus on application of digital pressure
- fistulous tract can be felt as a subcutaneous cord between the opening and the anal canal.

A5 Goodsall's rule states that for fistulous openings anterior to an imaginary transverse mid-anal line, the fistulous tract runs radially into the anal canal. For openings posterior to this line, the tract opens in the posterior midline of the anal canal.
    The exception to Goodsall's rule is the anterior opening, which is 3 cm or more from the anal verge, as this may be 'horse-shoeing' round from the posterior midline.

A6 Diagnosis:
- clinical examination
- examination under anaesthesia
- for suspected high/complex/recurrent fistula-in-ano – MRI scan.

Management:
- low fistula-in-ano – laying open of fistula (fistulotomy)
- high/complex fistula-in-ano – a seton (non-absorbable suture material) can be

threaded along the tract and loosely secured. It acts by slowly cutting through the tract and at the same time healing (fibrosis) takes place and hence the tract ultimately obliterates. The other options are anal plugs and anal flaps.

 The specific causes of fistula-in-ano are:
- Crohn's disease
- tuberculosis
- HIV infection
- colloid carcinoma of anal canal.

Your revision notes

Case 15

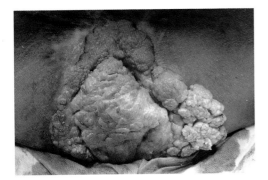

Figure 3.15a

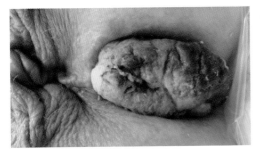

Figure 3.15b

Questions

(Q1) Figures 3.15a and 3.15b represent the same anal condition. What is the most likely diagnosis and what is the most common type?

(Q2) What is the aetiology of the most common type?

(Q3) How do you classify this problem?

(Q4) What are the clinical features?

(Q5) What is the mode of spread?

(Q6) How do you make a diagnosis and stage the disease?

(Q7) What are the treatment options?

Answers

(A1)   The most likely diagnosis is an anal canal cancer, most likely a squamous cell carcinoma.

(A2)
- Human Papilloma Virus (HPV) – perianal warts, Anal Intraepithelial Neoplasia (AIN) – majority of cases.
- HIV (Human Immunodeficiency Virus) infection.
- Immunosuppression.

(A3)   Anal canal cancers can be classified as follows:
- epidermoid carcinoma
- adenocarcinoma
- malignant melanoma.

Epidermoid carcinoma can be further histologically classified as follows:
- squamous cell carcinoma
- basaloid (cloacogenic) or mucoepidermoid carcinoma – junctional cancer arising from the dentate line where the squamous and glandular epithelium meets.

(A4)   Patients with anal canal cancer usually present with:
- symptoms:
  - perianal pain
  - bleeding
  - perianal itching
  - anal incontinence (locally advanced cases)
- signs:
  - malignant ulcer or growth at the anal margin or within the anal canal
  - enlarged inguinal lymph nodes

(A5)   Anal canal cancers can spread:
- locally:
  - proximally to rectum
  - laterally to anal sphincters
  - superiorly into the vagina
- locoregionally: lymphatic spread to perirectal and inguinal lymph nodes
- distant metastasis to liver, lung and bones.

(A6)   Diagnosis: biopsy of the anal lesion.
Staging:
- examination under anaesthetic to assess the local spread and to identify the sphincter involvement
- clinical examination of inguinal region for lymphadenopathy and fine needle aspiration cytology (FNAC) of the enlarged nodes
- MRI scan: to assess the locoregional involvement accurately
- CT scan: to assess the distant spread to liver, lungs.

Treatment options:
- small lesions at the anal margin: wide local excision
- larger lesions: radiotherapy + chemotherapy (5-FU + Mitomycin) – Nigro regimen
- recurrent lesions or poor response to chemo-irradiation: abdomino-perineal resection
- inguinal lymph node metastasis: radiotherapy or groin dissection.

Your revision notes

Case 16

This patient was noted to have discharged faecal fluid and flatus through his wound.

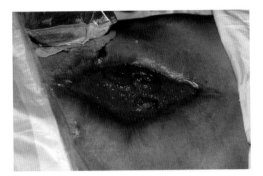

Figure 3.16

Questions

(Q1) What is the diagnosis?

(Q2) What is the definition of this condition?

(Q3) What are the possible causes for this?

(Q4) How can you classify the anatomical locations of this problem?

(Q5) What investigations would you instigate?

(Q6) What are the principles of treatment?

Answers

(A1) Postoperative faecal fistula (enterocutaneous fistula).

(A2) A fistula is an abnormal communication between two epithelial surfaces.
An enterocutaneous fistula is an abnormal connection between the GI tract and the skin.

(A3) Inflammation:
- inflammatory bowel disease especially Crohn's disease
- diverticulitis
- Tuberculosis.

Malignancy:
- following spontaneous rupture and abscess formation by the tumour.

Radiotherapy:
- pelvic irradiation can damage bowel.

Trauma:
- penetrating wounds to the abdomen. Perforation of loops of bowel can cause contamination and sepsis and fistulae formation.

Post-surgery:
- anastomotic leak especially in presence of sepsis or distal obstruction.

(A4) High versus low:
- high fistula (>500 ml/24 hrs) would involve stomach, duodenum, jejunum and ileum
- low fistula (<500 ml/24 hrs) involves large bowel. Fluid losses normally lower in this problem.

(A5) Blood tests:
- FBC – anaemia may be caused by sepsis and haemorrhage
- urea and electrolytes – patient can lose a lot of fluid through high fistulae and become hypokalaemic
- CRP + ESR
- blood cultures prior to commencement of antibiotics
- LFT – low albumin signifies malnutrition.

Radiological investigations – dependent on site:
- water soluble contrast follow through or enema
- fistulogram with screening to define anatomy of fistula
- MRI/CT to determine the extent of the cavity and detect underlying pathologies.

(A6) Early recourse to surgery especially in high intestinal fistulae, but high risk.
- Patients are fluid- and nutritionally depleted via the fistula – therefore require feeding parenterally and also strict input and output.
- Control sepsis with antibiotics.
- Relieve distal obstruction.
- Use of stoma adhesive around fistula site prevents enzyme-containing effluent from reaching and digesting skin around the fistula.
- If this is done 60% will heal at one month.

Case 17

A 43-year-old lady presented with sudden onset of acute colicky abdominal pain and distension and symptoms of constipation. On examination, there was gross abdominal distension with minimal tenderness. She had had a previous open hysterectomy and a bout of diarrhoea in the past week put down to food poisoning. Plain abdominal X-ray is shown in Figure 3.17a and a CT axial slice is shown in Figure 3.17b.

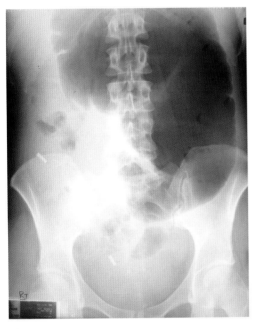

Questions

Q1 What is the most likely diagnosis? What sign is being demonstrated in Figure 3.17b?

Q2 What are the aetiological and risk factors for developing this condition?

Q3 Name other sites where this type of condition can occur.

Q4 What are the common complications of this condition?

Q5 Describe the treatment options.

Figure 3.17a

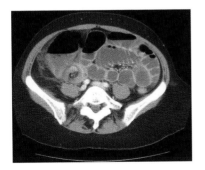

Figure 3.17b

Answers

 A1 Caecal volvulus.

Figure 3.17b: Whirl sign.

Plain abdominal X-ray is diagnostic in caecal volvulus in only about 50% of patients – typically a 'coffee bean' appearance directed towards the left upper quadrant. An inconclusive abdominal X-ray should prompt use of computerised tomogram with three-dimensional reconstruction or water-soluble enema. The use of barium is discouraged because of risk of peritonitis in case of bowel perforation.

A2 It occurs when there is congenital failure of fusion of peritoneum and ascending colon leading to a hypermobile caecum. Risk factors implicated in the aetiology are a high-fibre diet with consequent voluminous gas production, previous abdominal operations, increased peristalsis caused by diarrhoea, and distension by a distal obstruction. It is a closed loop obstruction that results from an axial rotation of the bowel upon its mesentery. It is more common in females.

A3 Gastric volvulus.
Small bowel volvulus – volvulus neonatorum.
Colon:
- sigmoid volvulus
- transverse colon
- splenic flexure (very rare).

Von Rokitansky first described colonic volvulus in 1836. Colonic volvulus constitutes 3–5% of all intestinal obstructions in the Western world. Sigmoid volvulus is the commonest constituting 40–80%, followed by caecal volvulus. Common symptoms are sudden onset of colicky abdominal pain, distension, absolute constipation and occasional vomiting. Signs are abdominal distension, a visible or palpable abdominal mass and minimal tenderness (signs of peritonitis may be noted with perforation).

A4 Obstruction.
Ischaemic bowel.
Necrosis and gangrene of the bowel.
Perforation.
Recurrence after resection.

Colonic volvulus is a life threatening condition. Mortality rates are:
- caecal volvulus – 10%
- sigmoid volvulus – 20%.

A5 Colonoscopic derotation:
Recommended in an acute setting and in the absence of clinical, laboratory or radiological signs of bowel necrosis or perforation. However the success varies. It is successful only in 50–60% in sigmoid volvulus and 10–20% in caecal volvulus. If successful a semi-elective single stage colonic resection can be done.

Gangrenous bowel is encountered in caecal volvulus in 20% of patients.

Surgical operations commonly performed are:
- resections
  - one-stage resection
  right hemicolectomy and primary ileo-colic anastomosis
  - two-stage resection.

If there is perforation and peritoneal soiling, a primary anastomosis is inadvisable and temporary ileostomy with colon as a mucus fistula is fashioned and further semi-elective procedure can be carried out for an anastomosis.
- Non-resectional techniques can be considered as a minimal procedure in high risk patients. However they are associated with high recurrence rates.
  - Simple derotation.
  - Caecostomy with caecopexy.
  - Caecopexy only.

Your revision notes

Case 18

This patient coughed 10 days post laparotomy for sigmoid colectomy. The nurses call you to see this frightening sight (Figure 3.18a).

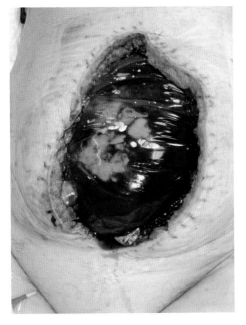

Figure 3.18a

Questions

Q1   What is the diagnosis?

Q2   Is there a warning sign that could have alerted the nurse or doctor that this was about to occur?

Q3   What are the predisposing factors that could lead to this condition?

Q4   What is your immediate management? What has the doctor done in Figure 3.18b? Is this correct?

Q5   What is the patient likely to develop?

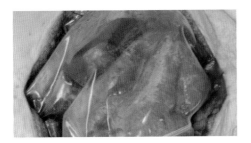

Figure 3.18b

Answers

(A1) Abdominal wound dehiscence.

(A2) The 'Pink Fluid' sign – serous blood-tinged fluid may ooze through the wound for several days before the actual dehiscence occurs.

(A3) Classify factors as preoperative, operative and postoperative.
- Preoperative: factors that affect wound healing include uraemia from CRF, protein deficiency, vitamin C deficiency or chronic cough (COPD).
- Operative: poor surgical technique during mass closure.
- Postoperative: abdominal distension, wound infection or haematoma.

(A4) Potential surgical emergency.
- Reassure patient and give opiate analgesia.
- Cover wound with saline-soaked sterile gauze (otherwise bowel will dry out and increase chance of postoperative ileus) – Figure 3.18 – wrong dressing but right idea with covering wound.
- Arrange theatre for immediate resuturing.

(A5) Paralytic ileus associated with other co-morbidities.

Section 4

Urology

Case I

A 65-year-old male presented with microscopic haematuria and right loin pain. He underwent a CT scan of his abdomen and pelvis.

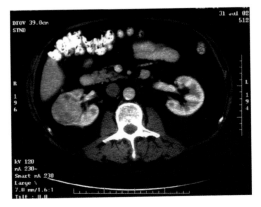

Figure 4.1

Questions

Q1 Describe the findings in Figure 4.1 and the possible diagnosis.

Q2 How would you treat this patient?

Q3 Name some inherited forms of this condition?

Q4 Give some indications for nephron-sparing surgery?

Q5 Name some histological subtypes of this condition?

Answers

(A1) The CT scan shows 5 cm solid tumour arising from the upper pole of the right kidney consistent with a likely diagnosis of renal cell carcinoma. The renal vein, hilar lymph nodes and inferior vena cava are clear of disease. The opposite kidney is normal in terms of size of parenchyma, suggestive that renal function will be normal after nephrectomy.

(A2) Right radical nephrectomy. The procedure can be done through a retroperitoneal (loin) or transabdominal approach. For very large tumours, a transabdominal approach has the advantage of providing adequate space for mobilization to dissect out the hilar vessels. Where expertise is available, the procedure should be done laparoscopically, and if anatomy is favourable (in terms of tumour clearance from the hilar vessels) then a partial nephrectomy is ideal to preserve nephrons. A partial nephrectomy can be done by open or laparoscopical measures, depending on the local expertise of the centre.

(A3) There are four well described types:
- Von Hippel–Lindau (VHL)
- hereditary papillary renal carcinoma (HPRC)
- hereditary leiomyoma renal cell carcinoma (HLRCC)
- Birt–Hogg–Dubé syndrome (BHD). BHD is a hereditary cancer and the affected individuals can have renal tumours, fibrofolliculomas and pulmonary cysts.

(A4) There are some absolute and relative indications for nephron-sparing surgery.
- Absolute indications:
  - tumour in anatomically or functionally solitary kidney
  - bilateral synchronous solid renal tumours.
- Relative indications:
  - selected patients with solid renal mass where contralateral kidney is threatened by local, systemic or genetic conditions that may affect the future renal function, e.g. diabetes, hypertension
  - likelihood of contralateral tumours (hereditary forms of renal cell carcinoma)
  - contralateral normal kidney where tumour size <4 cm (although this size is not absolute)
  - patient preference.

(A5) The various histological subtypes of primary renal cell cancers are:
- classical clear cell (arising from the proximal convoluted tubule)
- papillary (arising from the distal convoluted tubule)
- chromophobe (arising from the cortical portion of the collecting duct)
- collecting duct (very rare, usually in younger patients and carries a poor progosis)
- neuroendocrine
- medullary (arising from the calyceal epithelium, occurs in young, black sickle-cell sufferers and also carries a poor prognosis)
- unclassified.

Case 2

A 45-year-old female had an ultrasound for left loin discomfort. A left renal tumour was found. She subsequently had a CT scan.

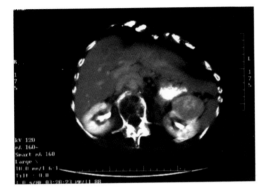

Figure 4.2

Questions

Q1 Describe the findings in Figure 4.2 and the possible differential diagnosis.

Q2 What are the radiological appearances of these conditions?

Q3 How are these conditions treated?

Answers

(A1) There is a 5 cm mass in the anterior aspect of the left kidney suggestive of a renal cell carcinoma (RCC). The possible differentials could be benign renal tumours like an oncocytoma or angiomyolipoma.

Oncocytoma is a benign renal tumour with rare malignant potential. It comprises 3–7% of renal tumours. Men are affected twice as commonly as women. It can occur concurrently with RCC or can mimic RCC radiologically. They may exhibit a classical spoke-wheel sign on CT due to the central stellate scar, but this may also occur in RCC.

Angiomyolipoma is a rare benign tumour of the kidney accounting for 0.3% of all renal neoplasms. It is seen in two distinct groups. It is found in 45–80% of patients with tuberous sclerosis, where tumours are typically bilateral and asymptomatic. Sporadic cases are commonly unilateral and tend to be larger than those associated with tuberous sclerosis.

(A2) The radiographic appearance is determined by the fat content. With ultrasound, tumours appear as well-circumscribed, echogenic and hyperechoic masses. The fat on CT scan appears black and measures –10 to –30 Houndsfield units. Negative Hounsfield units suggest the diagnosis of an angiomyolipoma.

(A3) Angiomyolipoma.

The treatment depends on the size and the symptoms. Nearly 80% of tumours <4 cm are asymptomatic. These can be followed with yearly imaging. Lesions larger than 4 cm with moderate or severe symptoms like bleeding or pain should undergo renal-sparing surgery or arterial embolisation.

Oncocytoma – total nephrectomy as pre-operatively they can be impossible to distinguish from RCC, which may also co-exist.

Case 3

A 45-year-old female developed persistent right loin pain. The CT scan is shown in Figure 4.3.

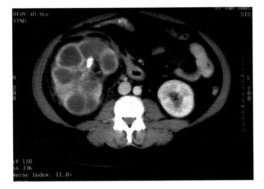

Figure 4.3

Questions

Q1 Describe the findings on the CT scan.

Q2 Explain the underlying pathology of this condition.

Q3 What is the clinical presentation of this condition?

Q4 How would you manage this patient?

Q5 What is emphysematous pyelonephritis?

Answers

(A1) The CT scan shows a right kidney with a staghorn calculus in the renal pelvis. There is a thin rim of enhancing parenchyma. The renal fascia is inflamed and thickened with perinephric stranding. The features are those of xanthogranulomatous pyelonephritis.

(A2) Xanthogranulomatous pyelonephritis is as a result of chronic bacterial infection of the kidney. Mostly occurs unilaterally. Severe inflammation and necrosis obliterates the renal parenchyma. Histology is characterised by the presence of lipid-laden histiocytes (xanthoma cells).

(A3) Patients commonly present with flank pain, fever, rigors and persistent bacteriuria. On physical examination, a flank mass can be palpable. *E. coli* or *Proteus* species are commonly cultured from the urine.

(A4) Right nephrectomy, ideally open as it is quite inflamed with obliteration of normal planes due the extensive inflammatory changes. Nephrectomy can be technically more difficult with higher complication rates. During the follow up, patients with recurrent stones may need to have metabolic evaluation to identify the risk of future renal stone formation, although staghorn stones are secondary to recurrent infection by urea splitting organisms and as such do not necessitate a full metabolic stone evaluation.

(A5) It is a necrotising infection of the kidney characterised by the presence of gas within the renal parenchyma or perinephric tissue. Risk factors include diabetes, where a high glucose content can allow the usual organisms (*E. Coli*, *Proteus* or *Klebsiella*) to ferment the glucose to produce carbon dioxide. Mortality in this condition is high and needs urgent treatment.

Case 4

A 70-year-old male presented with frank haematuria. The renal function and haematology results were within normal limits. An intravenous urogram (IVU) was requested followed by an MRI scan.

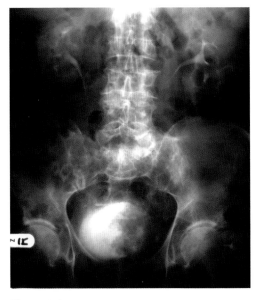

Figure 4.4a

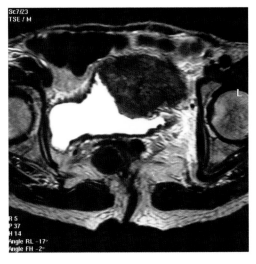

Figure 4.4b

Questions

Q1 Describe the findings and the most likely diagnosis.

Q2 What investigations should be undertaken in a patient presenting with haematuria?

Q3 How do you classify bladder tumours?

Q4 What are the risk factors for developing this disease?

Q5 How do you stage the condition?

Q6 What are the principles of management?

Q7 How are these patients followed up?

Answers

(A1) The IVU (Figure 4.4a) shows a filling defect on the left side of the bladder. Both kidneys are normal with no evidence of obstruction.

The MRI scan (Figure 4.4b) is a T_2-weighted image (water appears white) and reveals a large (approximately 10 cm) homogeneous mass invading the anterolateral wall of the bladder.

The most likely diagnosis is transitional cell carcinoma of bladder (TCC).

The differential diagnosis for filling defects in the bladder is a large blood clot, tumour and fungal ball.

(A2) The most commonly performed investigations are:
- urine microscopy, culture and sensitivity
- urine cytology
- cystoscopy
- renal tract ultrasound scan.

(A3) Bladder tumours can be classified as primary and secondary tumours.
- Primary:
  - transitional cell carcinoma (>90%)
  - squamous cell carcinoma (5–10%)
  - adenocarcinoma (2%)
  - undifferentiated carcinomas
  - mixed tumours.
- Secondary:
  - local invasion.

(A4) The risk factors for developing bladder cancer are:
- cigarette smoking
- occupational exposure to aniline dyes and aromatic amines (e.g. rubber and dye industries)
- Phenacetin abuse
- Cyclophosphamide chemotherapy.

(A5) Ta – confined to mucosa.
T_1 – invasion into lamina propria.
Tis – carcinoma in situ.
T_2a – invading superficial muscle.
T_2b – invading deep muscle.
T_3a – microscopic invasion of perivesical tissue.
T_3b – macroscopic invasion of perivesical tissue.
T_4a – invasion of prostate, uterus, vagina.
T_4b – invasion of pelvic side wall and abdominal wall.

(A6) The therapeutic options available are:
- non-invasive bladder cancer: endoscopic resection +/- intravesical chemo- or immunotherapy

- invasive bladder cancer: radical cystectomy or radical radiotherapy (still subject to debate)
- transurethral resection of the bladder tumour (TURBT). The procedure is done through a cystoscope. Bimanual examination provides useful information regarding the extent of the tumour. Intravesical mitomycin within the first 24 hours is a standard practice to help reduce the number of recurrences for superficial tumours (up to and including T_1 only).

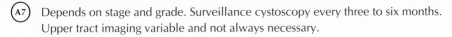 Depends on stage and grade. Surveillance cystoscopy every three to six months. Upper tract imaging variable and not always necessary.

Your revision notes

Case 5

This specimen was removed via a cystoscope in a 65-year-old male.

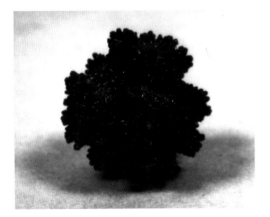

Figure 4.5

Questions

(Q1) Identify the specimen and explain why it is this colour.

(Q2) How are bladder stones classified?

(Q3) What factors predispose to the formation of bladder calculi?

(Q4) What is the classical triad of symptoms produced by a bladder stone?

(Q5) What investigations would confirm the diagnosis of a bladder stone?

Answers

(A1) The specimen shown is a sharp, spiky bladder calculus.

A calculus is a mass of precipitated solid material in a duct or an organ. The spiky appearance of this calculus is typical of calcium oxalate composition. Oxalate stones are normally white. However this stone is black due to blood pigment deposited on its rough surface as it traumatised the uroepithelium.

(A2) Bladder calculi can be classified as primary and secondary.
- Primary – made up of urate, oxalate, cystine or xanthine owing to an excess of these metabolites in the urine as a result of metabolic abnormalities.
- Secondary – made up of calcium and magnesium ammonium phosphate (triple phosphate) stone.

(A3) Factors predisposing the formation of bladder calculi are:
- anatomical abnormalities – cause stasis in the system or reflux. Examples include a duplex system, urethral valves in newborns and a horseshoe kidney
- stasis – pelviureteric junction obstruction
- infection – especially by *Proteus* species which are urea-splitting organisms that cause an alkaline urine resulting in precipitation and calculus formation
- increased concentration of calcium ions, e.g. in hyperparathyroidism – causes both nephrocalcinosis and calculus formation.

(A4) Urinary frequency, dysuria and haematuria.

(A5) Investigations:
- plain X-ray of KUB (kidneys, ureters, bladder): will invariably demonstrate the stone because of its high calcium content
- cystoscopy: will aid visualisation
- CT urogram: most sensitive investigation for the diagnosis of urinary tract calculi.

Case 6

A 40-year-old male presented to the urological outpatient clinic with this painless scrotal swelling.

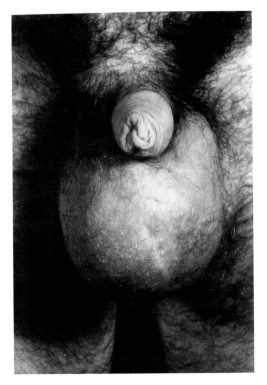

Questions

Q1 What is the most likely diagnosis?

Q2 What clinical findings would make you suspect this diagnosis?

Q3 Give a definition of this condition.

Q4 How is it classified?

Q5 Is ultrasound useful in the routine assessment of this problem?

Q6 What are the treatment options?

Q7 What is the main complication following surgical repair?

Figure 4.6

Answers

(A1) Hydrocoele.

(A2) Hydrocoele is usually a slowly and uniformly enlarging painless swelling confined to the scrotum with the underlying testis often not palpable through the tense swelling. The swelling is normally firm (tense or lax), non-tender and transilluminates. One can easily get above the swelling.

(A3) A hydrocoele is an abnormal collection of serous fluid within the tunica vaginalis of the testis, which forms the outer covering of the testis.

(A4) Hydrocoele can be classified on the basis of aetiology and types.
Aetiology: primary and secondary.
- Primary: idiopathic. Appears gradually and becomes large and tense – in children and the elderly.
- Secondary: associated with underlying testicular pathology. Appears rapidly, together with other symptoms.
- Underlying pathologies include:
  - trauma
  - tumour
  - torsion
  - epididymo-orchitis
  - following inguinal hernia repair
  - lymphatic obstruction.

Type: depends on which part of the processus vaginalis remains patent.
- Vaginal hydrocoele: most common type. Processus vaginalis is obliterated and the fluid collects only around the testicle.
- Congenital: the processus remains patent into the peritoneal cavity. Seen in infants. Usually resolves within the first 6–12 months of life but needs surgery if persists after a year.
- Infantile: rare. Processus obliterated at or near the deep inguinal ring but remains patent in the cord and scrotum. Thus the fluid accumulates around the cord as well as around the testicle.
- Hydrocoele of the cord: rarest. Fluid collection is around the cord only. Thus unlike other hydrocoeles, the testicle can be felt separately.

(A5) Diagnosis of a hydrocoele is usually clinical and rarely requires an ultrasound scan. However in suspicious cases and in cases of secondary hydrocoele, ultrasound scan can be performed to exclude testicular tumours and identify other underlying causes.

(A6) The treatment options can be classified as:
- non-surgical:
  - watchful waiting: if an underlying malignancy has been excluded clinically and with USS, it is reasonable to reassure patient and not operate for asymptomatic, small hydrocoeles.

- surgical:
    - Jaboulay's procedure: the sac is everted and approximated behind the cord via a longitudinal incision
    - Lord's plication: the sac is plicated with a series of interrupted stitches to the junction of the testis and epididymis.

(A7) The main complication following surgical repair for hydrocoele is haematoma formation. Therefore meticulous haemostasis is essential during the procedure. Later it may recur especially if it was large, in which case a Lord's plication may be warranted over a Jaboulay's procedure.

Your revision notes

Case 7

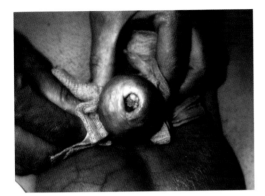

Figure 4.7a

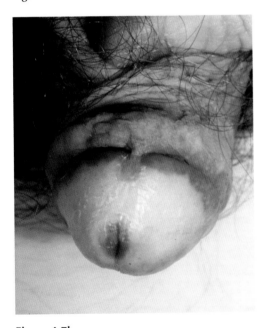

Figure 4.7b

Questions

(Q1) Identify the clinical condition shown in Figure 4.7a.

(Q2) What is the aetiology of this condition? What is the diagnosis in Figure 4.7b?

(Q3) What is the natural history of the prepuce and its function in children?

(Q4) What are the complications of this condition?

(Q5) What is the surgical management and its complications?

(Q6) What is meant by a paraphimosis and how will you manage it?

Answers

(A1) Phimosis: gross narrowing of the preputial orifice. Due to the white scarring of the foreskin, it can be said to be secondary to Balanitis Xerotica Obliterans (BXO).

(A2) The various causes for the development of phimosis are:
- children: congenital/physiological phimosis and scarring due to recurrent balanoprosthitis. BXO may also be a cause
- adult men: balanitis xerotica obliterans (Figure 4.7b).
- elderly: chronic balanitis, most likely associated with diabetes.

(A3) At birth the prepuce is normally adherent to the glans and therefore non-retractile. By puberty it is fully retracted in most boys.

   The prepuce is thought to protect the glans and urethral orifice from the excoriation of ammoniacal dermatitis.

(A4) Infection can lead to scarring and fibrosis of the prepuce with consequent narrowing of the orifice. However, in most cases of BXO no preceding history of recurrent infections or inflammation is obtained.

(A5) Management:
- it is important, particularly in children to distinguish physiological from pathological phimosis. Physiological phimosis is to be managed with reassurance and education to the parents, although in some cases topical steroids may be used
- in children, sometimes just the preputial adhesions need to be divided
- true pathological phimosis is best treated with circumcision
- risks/complications of circumcision include infection, bleeding/haematoma, excision of too much skin, injury to the glans penis, breakdown of the wound and in meatal stenosis from extension of BXO scarring to involve the meatus and distal urethra.

(A6) Paraphimosis occurs when a tight prepuce is retracted and fails to return. If it is not subsequently pushed back, the constriction leads to oedema of the glans, pain and occasionally necrosis. This condition needs to be avoided after male catheterisation.

   Treatment: manual replacement using gentle pressure with or without local anaesthesia using a penile block. If this is not possible, dorsal slit and then later circumcision after inflammation has settled allowing normal tissue planes and anatomy to be restored.

Case 8

This shows the cut section of a testis which was removed from a 22-year-old male.

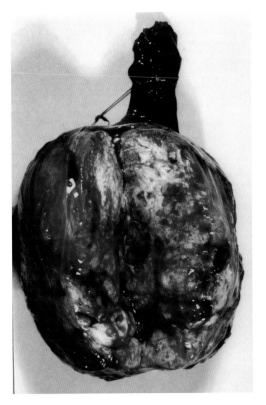

Figure 4.8

Questions

(Q1) What is the most likely diagnosis and why?

(Q2) What are the clinical features of this disease?

(Q3) What is the differential diagnosis?

(Q4) What is the mode of spread?

(Q5) How do you investigate and stage this?

(Q6) What are the treatment options?

Answers

 The diagnosis is malignant teratoma of the testis (Non-semonomatous Germ Cell tumour – NSGCT).

Grossly the specimen shows areas of solid and cystic tissue. Testicular teratoma tends to occur in the younger age group, the peak incidence being 20–30 years. The differential diagnosis is a seminoma of the testis.

Teratoma arises from the totipotent cells in the testis and often contains a variety of cells which may be ecto- or mesodermal in origin. Nodules of cartilage, hair, bone, etc. may be present. Previously was classified on the basis of differentiation as:
- differentiated teratoma
- malignant teratoma intermediate – most common
- undifferentiated or anaplastic teratoma
- malignant teratoma trophoblastic – uncommon.

Seminoma is the commonest testicular tumour and is commoner between the ages of 35 and 45 years. The enlarged testis is smooth and firm. The cut surface is homogeneous and pinkish cream in colour. Histologically there are sheets of oval cells separated by a fine fibrous stroma.

 Symptoms:
- testicular swelling
- sensation of heaviness
- only 10% experience pain
- rarely, may present from metastases to lymph nodes (abdominal mass), lung (haemoptysis, cough), brain (confusion, headaches), bone or liver.

Signs:
- solid scrotal mass which is firm and attached to the testis, but does not transluminate
- may have a secondary hydrocoele.

 The differential diagnosis of testicular tumours includes:
- epididymo-orchitis
- hydrocoele or tense epididymal cyst
- torsion
- syphilitic gumma
- granulomatous/tuberculous orchitis.

(A4) Testicular tumours usually spread via haematogenous or lymphatic route.
- Teratoma spreads by haematogenous route commonly, but also spreads by lymphatics. Pulmonary metastasis may suggest a teratoma.
- Seminoma mainly spreads by lymphatics, whereas haematogenous route is less common. Occasionally, an enlarged supraclavicular lymph node may be the presenting sign.

Lymphatic spread initially involves para-aortic lymph nodes, and later the supra-diaphragmatic or supra-clavicular lymph nodes.

Every patient presenting with a testicular swelling must be carefully assessed with the possibility of tumour in mind.

Preliminary ultrasound of the scrotum may be helpful, especially where the testis is not palpable in cases of a large hydrocoele.

Staging investigations should not delay orchidectomy.

Staging investigations include:

- radioimmunoassay for tumour markers – human chorionic gonadotrophin (hCG), alpha feto protein (AFP) and lactate dehydrogenase (LDH) – they help to diagnose, and to assess the effectiveness of treatment
- CT chest, abdomen and pelvis and MRI – to detect secondaries and also to detect response to treatment
- histological analysis of the tumour (high orchidectomy/inguinal approach for orchidectomy with early dissection and soft clamping of the cord prior to delivery of the testis).

hCG levels are raised in 30% of seminomas and 40% of teratomas, but AFP elevation indicates a teratomatous element.

Staging of testicular tumours:

stage 1: testis lesion only – no spread

stage 2: nodes below the diaphragm only

stage 3: nodes above the diaphragm

stage 4: visceral (pulmonary and liver) metastasis.

 Treatment options:

- teratoma: not radiosensitive:
  - stage 1 can be managed by either chemotherapy to treat the 20% of patients who may have occult micrometastases to para-aortic lymoh nodes or surveillance by regular tumour markers and CT scans on the basis that treating all patients with chemotherapy to target the 20% of these patients that may have micrometastasis is probably over-kill
  - stages 2–4 can be treated with chemotherapy. Ideally BEP – bleomycin, etopside and Cisplatin, although methotrexate, and vincristine have been used especially as second or third line with good results.
- seminoma: radiosensitive:
  - radiotherapy was the mainstay of treatment in stage 1 and 2 disease. More recently trials have shown that for stage 1 disease, 1 dose of carboplatin is as effective as radiotherapy to para-aortic nodes. BEP is still used for stage 2 disease
  - stages 3 and 4 are treated with chemotherapy.

Retroperitoneal lymph node dissection is sometimes needed if the masses remain after chemotherapy especially for NSGCT.

Prognosis depends on the histological type and stage of the disease.

- Teratoma – In stage 1 and 2, the five-year survival is 85%. It drops to 60% in advanced disease.
- Seminoma – If there is no metastasis, 95% will be alive at five years after treatment. It drops to 75% with extensive visceral secondaries.

Your revision notes

Case 9

Figure 4.9 is from a 55-year-old male.

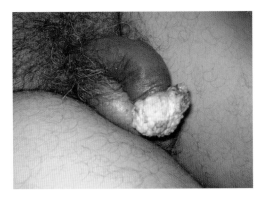

Figure 4.9

Questions

(Q1) What is the most likely diagnosis?

(Q2) What are the potential causes and predisposing factors?

(Q3) What pre-malignant changes are associated with this condition?

(Q4) What is the clinical course of this disease?

(Q5) What are the treatment options?

Answers

A1 Invasive squamous cell carcinoma of the penis.

A2 The causes and predisposing factors are:
- presence of a foreskin and poor hygiene – accumulation of carcinogens within smegma under the foreskin
- HPV 16 and 18
- smoking
- pre-malignant conditions, e.g. Bowen's disease or erythroplasia of Queyrat, Leukoplakia.

A3 The premalignant conditions of penile cancer are:
- leukoplakia
- erythroplasia of Queyrat (carcinoma in situ)
- cutaneous horn – overgrowth and cornification of the epithelium.

A4 Clinical course:
- typically presents as epithelial thickening of the glans or the inner surface of the prepuce progressing to ulcero-infiltrative or exophytic growth eroding the penile tip, shaft or both
- usually grows slowly with metastasis to the regional lymph nodes (inguinal and iliac)
- distant metastasis are uncommon especially if lymph nodes are clear
- five-year survival rate is 66% if lesion confined to penis, but only 27% with regional lymph node involvement.

A5 The treatment options available are radiotherapy, surgery and chemotherapy.
- Small localised lesions can be treated with external beam radiotherapy, topical treatment with 5FU or imiquimod.
- Large lesions can be treated with surgery:
  - glans resurfacing or glansectomy
  - partial penile amputation if at least 2 cm of residual penis length can be preserved after giving a reasonable margin clearance (used to be 2 cm, but now less is accepted)
  - total penile amputation with perineal urethrostomy can be performed.
- Ilioinguinal lymph node dissection can be performed in case of involved regional lymph nodes or in cases of higher local stage and grade.
- Fixed lymph nodes – palliative treatment with chemotherapy.
- Metastatic disease – chemotherapy.

Case 10

A 65-year-old male was admitted with sudden onset of right loin pain radiating to the groin. On examination, he was febrile and tachycardic. The white count was elevated. The X-ray of his abdomen is shown in Figure 4.10a.

A 55-year-old male was admitted with sudden onset of colicky right loin pain radiating to his groin. His abdomen was not peritonitic and his urine test is positive for microscopic haematuria. Figure 4.10b shows an unenhanced CT scan of his abdomen and pelvis.

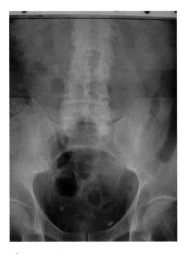

Figure 4.10a

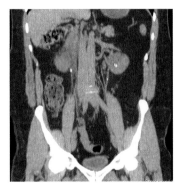

Figure 4.10b

Questions

(Q1) Describe the findings of Figure 4.10a and Figure 4.10b.

(Q2) Apart from an unenhanced CT scan, what investigation would be appropriate after a plain X-ray?

(Q3) What is the most appropriate clinical management of a patient with a dense nephrogram and complete obstruction on an IVU?

(Q4) What are the clinical features of renal colic?

(Q5) How would you confirm your diagnosis?

(Q6) How would you manage renal tract calculus disease?

(Q7) How do you classify renal stones?

(Q8) What is a struvite stone?

Answers

(A1) Plain X-ray (Figure 4.10a) shows a 1.5 cm stone in the right ureter adjacent to the transverse process of L3. Other calcific areas in the pelvis probably represent phleboliths. Phleboliths represents calcifications within the pelvic veins. They are rounder, lateral to the course of the ureter, and have radiolucent centres. A leaking abdominal aneurysm can also present like this. Careful clinical examination is very important. Sometimes a calcified aneurysm wall can be seen on the plain X-ray.

The CT scan image with reconstruction (Figure 4.10b) shows a 6 mm stone in the right upper ureter and a 5 mm stone in the left mid-ureter. Two stones are also seen in the left kidney. The diagnosis is renal colic.

(A2) An intravenous urogram. Some centres use CT scan as the gold standard in patients with renal colic. CT scan is more sensitive and specific than an IVU.

(A3) In an acute setting, ureteric stenting or nephrostomy is carried out as an emergency. Stone removal is carried out as a second stage. Most centres prefer extracorporeal shockwave lithotripsy (ESWL) for stones in the proximal ureter (above the iliac vessels). Distal ureters are managed with ureteroscopes. This man had an emergency stenting.

(A4) Symptoms:
- sudden onset colicky abdominal pain radiating from loin to groin, sometimes to the scrotum, tip of penis or labia, often associated with nausea and vomiting
- difficulty in micturition
- frequency and or urgency in micturition
- septic symptoms, haematuria.

Signs:
- patient cannot lie still due to pain
- urine analysis reveals microscopic haematuria (although the longer the history, the lower the likelihood of finding haematuria and so negative dipstick does not rule out renal colic).

Patients can also present with obstructive uropathy leading to:
- hydronephrosis
- pyonephrosis
- septicaemia
- end-stage renal failure secondary to bilateral renal calculus disease or in a solitary functioning kidney.

(A5) Other investigations:
- urinalysis will reveal microscopic haematuria
- plain abdominal X-ray reveals 90% of renal tract calculi
- CT-Urogram is the investigation of choice as it is extremely sensitive in identifying renal tract calculus. It can also reveal associated obstructive changes, e.g. pelvicaliceal dilatation, hydroureteronephrosis, perinephric stranding
- intravenous urogram and ultrasound can be performed but CT-Urogram is the investigation of choice.

Management depends on the following factors:
- size of the calculus
- site of the calculus
- presence of renal tract obstruction/infection
- renal function.

Initial management consists of adequate pain relief, and renal function assessment.
- Calculus less than 6 mm in size will pass on its own, especially if in distal ureter and only needs expectant management with analgesia and alpha receptor antagonists, which relax lower ureteric smooth muscle and has been shown in meta-analysis to increase stone passage rates.
- Calculus larger than 6 mm will need intervention, the timing of which depends on renal function, renal tract obstruction and sepsis.
- If renal function satisfactory and no obstruction or sepsis, patient can be managed conservatively initially, followed by early elective intervention in the form of ureteroscopic extraction or ureteric stenting and ESWL (Extracorporeal Shock Wave Lithotripsy).
- In cases of renal tract obstruction, sepsis, worsening renal function or patients with solitary kidney, emergent intervention is required in the form of percutaneous nephrostomy or ureteric stenting.

 Renal stones can be classified as:
- calcium oxalate stones (85%)
- struvite stones (infective or triple phosphate stones) in 15%
- uric acid stones (5–10%)
- cystine stones (1–5%) – inherited as autosomal recessive trait.

 Struvite stones are infectious stones made of calcium magnesium ammonium phosphate. They are more common in women (2:1). Alkaline urine caused by breakdown of urea (by urease produced by *Proteus*, *Pseudomonas* and *Klebsiella* spp.) paves way for the formation of these stones. A pH >7.0 is needed for stone formation. The stones can fill the entire renal collecting system (staghorn stones).

Your revision notes

Case 11

This 45-year-old male presented with several scrotal masses, which were separate from the testes and felt firm and loculated. Figure 4.11a shows the ultrasound of one of these masses.

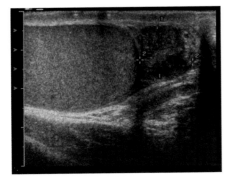

Figure 4.11a

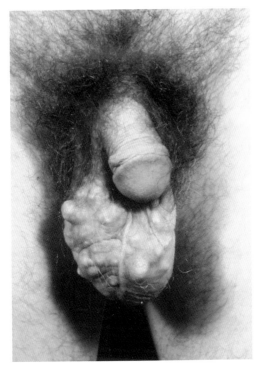

Figure 4.11b

Questions

(Q1) What is the most likely diagnosis?

(Q2) How are they caused?

(Q3) What are the defining features?

(Q4) What are the management options?

(Q5) What risks should you warn the patient about if they undergo removal?

(Q6) Look at Figure 4.11b. What is the spot diagnosis?

Answers

(A1) Multiple epididymal cysts.

(A2) Occasionally they occur as a complication of vasectomy. In these cases they are full of sperm and are termed spermatocoeles.

(A3) Mass(es) are often multiple and most commonly arise in the head of the epididymis – separate from the testis.
Firm and may be loculated.
Brilliantly transilluminable (classical) unless they contain sperm.
Separate from the superficial inguinal ring (can 'get above' mass(es)).

(A4) Non-surgical versus surgical.
- Non-surgical: if asymptomatic they should be left alone especially in younger males where there is a risk of subfertility if operated upon, since epididymal obstruction can occur. An alternative to surgical removal is aspiration, though recurrence is usual.
- Surgical: very large or painful cysts can be removed. Occasionally the whole of the epididymis is excised to prevent recurrence.

(A5) BAUS procedure specific consent form – recommended discussion of adverse events.
Occasional:
- recurrence of fluid collection can occur
- collection of blood around the testis – can resolve slowly or require surgical removal
- infection of incision or testis requiring further treatment.

Rare:
- scarring can damage the epididymis causing subfertility.

Alternative therapy:
- observation
- removal of fluid with a needle.

(A6) Multiple scrotal sebaceous cysts.

Case 12

A 60-year-old man presented to the GP with lower urinary tract symptoms. The PSA was 19.5. He underwent this investigation (Figure 4.12).

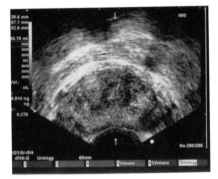

Figure 4.12

Questions

(Q1) What is the investigation? What are the possible complications of this procedure?

(Q2) What does it show? How is prostate cancer graded?

(Q3) Give the treatment options available.

(Q4) What are the indications to perform the prostate biopsy?

(Q5) Name a recent advance in managing this condition.

Answers

(A1) The picture shows a transrectal ultrasound of the prostate gland. Biopsies are taken under transrectal ultrasound guidance. The procedure is usually done under local anaesthesia. Complications of this procedure include haematuria, urinary retention, bleeding per rectum, haemospermia. Mortality secondary to sepsis has also been reported following this procedure.

(A2) TRUS shows a hypoechoic area in the peripheral zone of the prostate likely to represent a malignancy (prostate cancer).

Gleason grading.
It is based on the glandular pattern of the tumour as identified at relatively low magnification. Cytologic features play no role in the grade of the tumour. The primary (or the most predominant) and the secondary (or the second most prevalent) architectural patterns are assigned a grade from 1 to 5, with 1 the most differentiated and 5 the least differentiated. The total gives the Gleason score or the sum.

(A3) For localised disease:
- radical prostatectomy – open (retropubic or perineal) or minimally invasive (laparoscopic or robotic assisted)
- radical radiotherapy
- brachytherapy
- watchful waiting.

For locally advance or metastatic disease:
- hormone deprivation treatment.

(A4) Abnormal digital rectal examination.
PSA elevated more than the age specific range – PSA is a serine protease secreted by the prostatic epithelium.
Note false positive PSA elevation can occur in BPH, prostatitis, recent sexual activity.

(A5) Brachytherapy – interstitial radiotherapy used for managing organ-confined prostate cancer. Suitable for smaller prostate with low volume cancer in men with minimal lower tract symptoms.
Robotic prostatectomy.

Case 13

This 35-year-old male presents with intermittent right loin pain. On examination, he was afebrile with right loin tenderness. Plain X-ray abdomen did not reveal any renal stones. An IVU was requested (Figure 4.13).

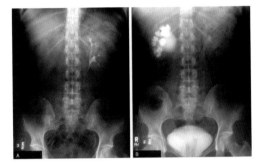

Figure 4.13

Questions

Q1   Describe the IVU findings and the diagnosis.

Q2   What further investigations are needed?

Q3   Name some complications of this condition.

Q4   How can this condition be treated?

Q5   Give some of the recent advances in managing this condition.

Answers

(A1) IVU shows dilatation of the right renal pelvis with a normal ureter in keeping with pelviureteric junction obstruction (PUJ). This condition is probably the most common congenital abnormality of the ureter, occurring more often in boys than in girls (5:2 ratio). It is more common on the left side (5:2) and can be bilateral in 10–15% of the cases.

(A2) Isotope renogram with Technetium-labelled mercapto acetyl guanine (MAG 3) to assess the degree of obstruction. Additional diagnostic tools include spiral CT, transluminal ultrasound, and Whitaker's test.

(A3) Recurrent UTI, stone formation, sepsis, loss of kidney function.

(A4) Anderson–Hynes dismembered pyeloplasty. The purpose of this procedure is to remove the narrowed portion of the PUJ and attach the ureter to the renal pelvis in a way that allows easy drainage of urine.

(A5) Laparoscopic pyeloplasty – non-randomised studies show equal efficacy with this procedure whilst avoiding the loin scar and reducing the hospital stay.

Endoscopic procedures:
- retrograde endopyelotomy
- balloon rupture
- antegrade endopyelotomy
- stent insertion (retrograde or antegrade) with six-monthly to yearly stent changes.

Case 14

A 15-year-old boy presented to A&E with a four-hour history of left-sided testicular pain. There was no history of systemic illness, testicular trauma or urinary symptoms. Examination revealed mild scrotal erythema, a high-riding and tender left testis.

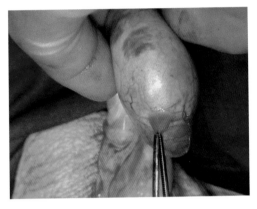

Figure 4.14

Questions

Q1 What is the most likely diagnosis and why? What is the differential diagnosis?

Q2 What investigations may be performed to support this diagnosis?

Q3 Figure 4.14 was taken during exploration of this boy's left testicle. What do you see?

Q4 How would you manage the patient?

Q5 Suppose that this patient in fact had only a torted hydatid cyst of Morgagni, would you explore the contralateral side?

Answers

 Most likely diagnosis is acute left testicular torsion.
Reasons:
- left testicle is higher than the right one ('high-riding'). Usually also lies in a horizontal plane. This is consistent with twisting and shortening of the spermatic cord
- testicular torsion can occur at any age, but most common in boys aged 13–17 (prevalence 1/125 males)
  - an abnormally high investment of the tunica vaginalis allows excess mobility of the testicle (the classical 'bell-clapper' deformity)
  - incomplete attachment of the testes to the epididymis allows it to rotate alone – less common
  - trauma and exercise can produce the cremasteric reflex. This can precede the torsion and some patients recount previous episodes of similar pain due to recurrent torsions that spontaneously resolve
- remember, patients with cryptorchidism are at increased risk of torsion and also young patients with abdominal pain should have their external genitalia examined for this condition.

Differential diagnosis:
- torsion of a hydatid cyst of Morgagni
- acute epididymo-orchitis (rare)
- strangulated inguinal hernia
- idiopathic scrotal oedema.

 None.
Diagnosis is made on clinical grounds. Urgent surgical exploration is required if there is any doubt about the diagnosis!
There is normally a time window of four to six hours from the onset of pain where testicular salvage is possible – after this the testicle has a much higher chance of loss. In some instances even a shorter delay leads to loss of the testicle; therefore speed in exploration is critical!

However:
- urinalysis – to exclude UTI causing epididymo-orchitis
- gray scale ultrasound – may show the affected testicle to be enlarged and hypoechoic. In contrast, in epididymitis the testis is normal
- colour Doppler ultrasonography – used to assess testicular blood flow. Sensitivity and specificity 95% (but operator dependent).

(A3) A torted left testicle (note the discolouration of the testicle).
Forceps is holding an incidental hydatid cyst of Morgagni, which is not torted.

(A4) Points to consider:
- informed consent for bilateral scrotal exploration, possible ipsilateral orchidectomy,

and contralateral orchidopexy should be obtained in all cases from parents and if appropriate the patient

- if testicular torsion, untwist spermatic cord and wrap testis in a warm saline soaked swab before deciding on its viability (for 10 minutes). Ask the anaesthetist to increase the ventilated oxygen!
- if viable after assessment, return testis to scrotum and suture to dartos muscle at three different points to prevent recurrence. The other testis is similarly fixated either through the same incision or a separate one
- if orchidectomy required – in order to prevent testicular gangrene or scrotal abscess or prevent the formation of anti-sperm antibodies that would render an adult with a single testis infertile – get a second opinion from your consultant
- if a torted hydatid cyst of Morgagni is found this is excised or diathermied and the testis is fixated. Similarly (testis fixation) if epididymo-orchitis found, except culture swab also taken and patient commenced on antibiotics
- in these two circumstances the testis is fixed to prevent diagnostic confusion in future if the boy represents with testicular pain.

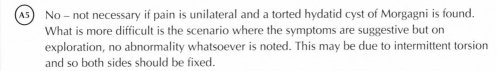 No – not necessary if pain is unilateral and a torted hydatid cyst of Morgagni is found. What is more difficult is the scenario where the symptoms are suggestive but on exploration, no abnormality whatsoever is noted. This may be due to intermittent torsion and so both sides should be fixed.

Radiology for the surgical trainee

Case 1

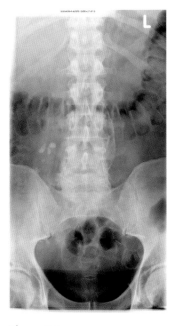

Figure 5.1a

Questions

(Q1) What is the most significant abnormality in the above radiographs (Figures 5.1a–d), and what is the diagnosis?

(Q2) What are the risk factors for developing this condition?

(Q3) What are the potential complications?

(Q4) What other method of imaging can be used to evaluate this further?

(Q5) What are the different types of this condition and which are the commonest?

(Q6) On ultrasound, when is an aorta considered aneurysmal?

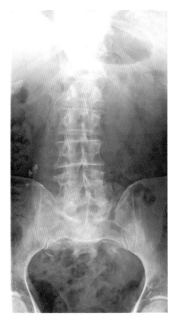

Figure 5.1b

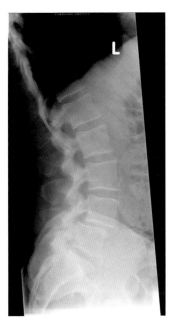

Figure 5.1c

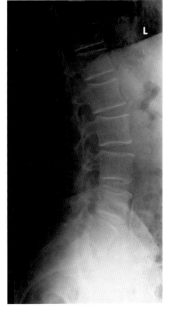

Figure 5.1d

Answers

(A1) Calcification is seen adjacent to the spine. This is a plain film sign of an abdominal aortic aneurysm.

(A2) Male sex, Caucasian ethnicity, >75 years of age, vascular disease, high blood pressure, smoking, family history, high cholesterol.

(A3) Rupture – 25%.
Peripheral embolisation.
Infection.
Occlusion of the aorta.

(A4) Computerised Tomography (CT)   Ultrasound

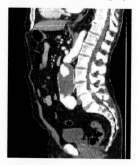

Figure 5.1e

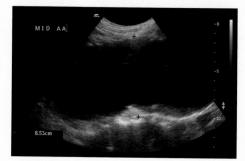

Figure 5.1f

(A5) True aneurysm: dilatation of all layers of the wall of the aorta, which is intact although weakened.

False aneurysm: all layers of the aortic wall are perforated. The leaking blood is contained by adventitia, connective tissue, etc.

Commonest:
• fusiform: circumferential dilatation of the aorta – 80%
• saccular: only a focal part of the wall is involved.

(A6) Diameter is >3 cm.

Case 2

A 27-year-old male with a two-day history of abdominal pain with vomiting and diarrhoea. The pain was central initially but moved to the right iliac fossa. On examination the patient was afebrile and the abdomen was distended. There was tenderness on the right side but no peritonism.

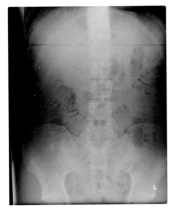

Figure 5.2a

Questions

Q1 What is the most likely diagnosis based on Figure 5.2a?

Q2 What feature on the X-ray supports this diagnosis? How confident is this diagnosis based on the information given so far? What is the patient at risk of?

Q3 If the patient suddenly developed a high temperature what would you suspect?

Q4 What other imaging modalities could be used to confirm the diagnosis?

Q5 What features of this condition are seen on CT (Figures 5.2b and c)?

Q6 What features of this condition are seen on ultrasound (Figures 5.2d and e)?

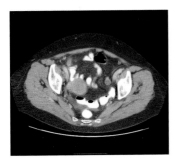

Figure 5.2b

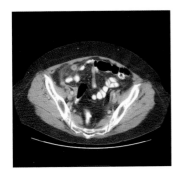

Figure 5.2c

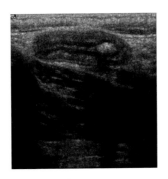

Figure 5.2d

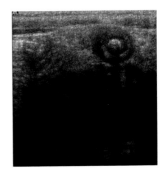

Figure 5.2e

Answers

(A1) Acute appendicitis.

(A2) A calcified appendicolith is visible in the right iliac fossa.

Abdominal pain with an appendicolith seen on plain film gives a 90% probability of appendicitis.

In acute appendicitis the presence of an appendicolith indicates a high risk for perforation and gangrene.

(A3) Normally in appendicitis the patient is afebrile or has a low-grade fever. If the fever rises above 38.5°C perforation should be suspected.

(A4) CT.
Ultrasound.

(A5) The appendix is identified as a blind-ended sac arising from the caecum in the right iliac fossa.

In appendicitis there is:
- a distended appendix lumen >7 mm in diameter
- circumferential enhancing wall thickening – target sign (Figure 5.2c)
- periappendicular inflammation – stranding of the adjacent fat.

(A6) Distended appendix >6 mm with mural wall thickness >2 mm.

Laminated wall giving the target appearance.

Appendix is non-compressible.

Appendicolith seen in the distal end of the appendix as a hyperechogenic focus with posterior acoustic shadowing.

Case 3

A 37-year-old female with right upper quadrant pain and bilious vomiting. On examination the patient's abdomen was distended and tender.

Her white cell count and C-reactive protein were raised.

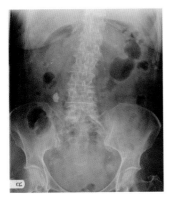

Figure 5.3a

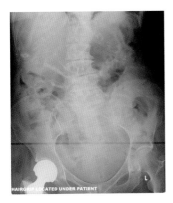

Figure 5.3b

Questions

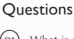

Q1   What is seen in Figure 5.3a?

Q2   What sign is seen in Figure 5.3b?

Q3   What is the most likely diagnosis?

Q4   What other examination should be requested?

Q5   What might this reveal?

Q6   Which is the odd one out of the three erect chest X-rays (Figures 5.3c–e), and why?

Q7   What do the other two films show?

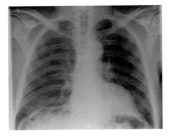

Figure 5.3c

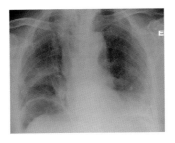

Figure 5.3d

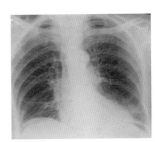

Figure 5.3e

Answers

(A1) Free gas is visible in the right upper quadrant.

(A2) Rigler's sign – This is when the bowel wall is clearly defined by gas on both the intra- and extraluminal sides of the bowel wall, due to the presence of free gas in the peritoneal cavity.

(A3) Perforated viscus causing free intraperitoneal gas.

(A4) Erect chest X-ray.

(A5) Free gas under the diaphragm.

(A6) Figure 5.3c.

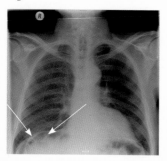

This is Chilaiditi's syndrome (*see* Figure 5.3f below) – there is a loop of bowel lying above the liver, NOT free air under the right hemidiaphragm. If you look carefully you can see the haustra of the bowel running almost vertically downwards!

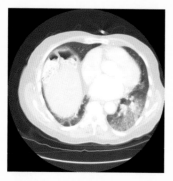

Figure 5.3f: Chilaiditi on CT

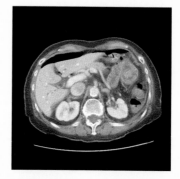

Figure 5.3g: Free gas on CT

(A7) Free gas under the diaphragm.

Case 4

A 70-year-old lady with shortness of breath and neck pain radiating to the chest. A CXR was performed (Figure 5.4a).

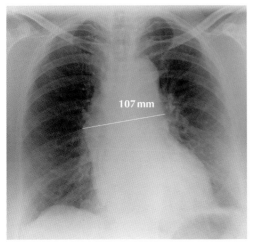

107 mm

Figure 5.4a

Questions

(Q1)   What mediastinal width is cause for concern?

(Q2)   What is the major concern and why?

(Q3)   What other plain film signs should be checked for (not seen in this X-ray)?

(Q4)   Does a normal chest X-ray exclude this diagnosis?

(Q5)   What imaging should be done next?

(Q6)   How is this condition classified?

(Q7)   What are the treatment options?

Answers

(A1) A superior mediastinal width of >80 mm.

(A2) Aortic dissection/rupture.
A widened superior mediastinal width may be due to an enlarging false channel or haematoma from a rupture.

(A3) Calcification sign – atherosclerotic plaque is displaced inwards by a false lumen, away from the true wall – only applies to the descending aorta.
Difference in size between the ascending and descending aorta.
Irregular aortic contour.
Cardiac enlargement.
Left pleural effusion.
Atelectasis.
Displacement of trachea to the right.

(A4) NO – 25% of chest X-rays will be normal.

(A5) CT of the aorta.
The dissection flap can clearly be seen in Figures 5.4b–d.

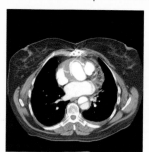 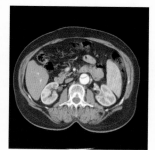 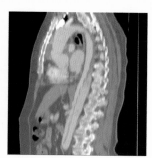

Figure 5.4b   **Figure 5.4c**   **Figure 5.4d**

(A6) Stanford classification is preferable to DeBakey as it guides treatment options.
- Type A – ascending aorta and arch affected (regardless of whether the descending aorta is involved).
- Type B – descending aorta only.

(A7) Type A – reinforcement of aortic wall with surgical graft.
Type B – medical treatment to reduce peak systolic blood pressure.

Case 5

An 85-year-old male from a nursing home, on long-term laxatives. He complains of abdominal pain. Bowels have not been opening. On examination the abdomen is distended and tender.

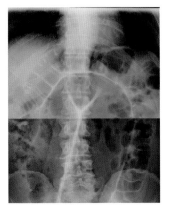

Figure 5.5a

Questions

(Q1)   What sign is seen in these X-rays?

(Q2)   What is the likely diagnosis?

(Q3)   What complications can occur if left untreated?

(Q4)   Which of the pictures shown here is the odd one out and why?

(Q5)   How can the two types be differentiated radiologically?

(Q6)   What are the typical patient populations of both types?

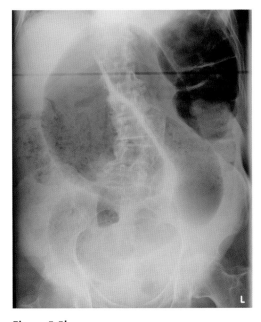

Figure 5.5b

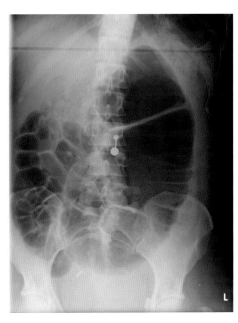

Figure 5.5c

Answers

(A1) Coffee bean sign – this is seen on supine films – twisting of the mesentery causes the appearance of a line between two distended gas-filled loops of bowel.

(A2) Colonic volvulus.

(A3) Perforation.
Infarction.
Abdominal compartment syndrome – increasing abdominal pressure causes decreased respiratory function and cardiac output.

(A4) Figure 5.5c – this is a caecal volvulus, the other two are sigmoid.

(A5) Sigmoid: may be large- and small-bowel gas-filled loops – no gas is seen distal to the sigmoid.
Caecal: gas-filled loop of small bowel may be seen, BUT NO gas-filled colon is seen distal to the caecum, unless the volvulus is intermittent or incomplete.

(A6) Sigmoid: elderly or mentally ill patients.
Caecal: the young adult (20–40) – males more than females.

Case 6

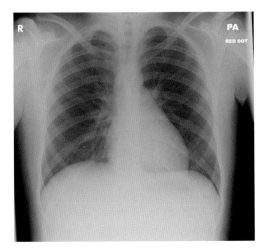

Figure 5.6a

Questions

(Q1) What is the abnormality seen in Figures 5.6a–c?

(Q2) Can you locate it in the large PA chest radiograph?

(Q3) Where do these commonly lodge and why?

(Q4) What are the dimensions that would cause concern about the object not passing?

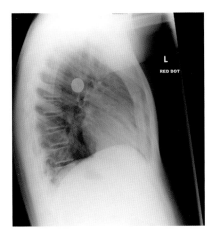

Figure 5.6b

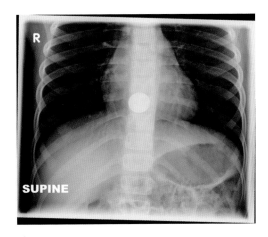

Figure 5.6c

Answers

(A1) Swallowed battery lodged within the oesophagus.

(A2)

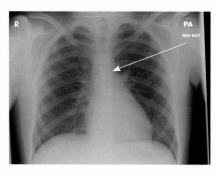

(A3) Thoracic inlet – where skeletal muscle changes to smooth muscle, and also the level of the cricopharyngeus sling at C6.
Mid oesophagus – where the aortic arch and carina indent the oesophagus.
The lower oesophageal sphincter at the gastro-oesophageal junction.

(A4) 6 cm long, 2 cm wide.
Other examples:

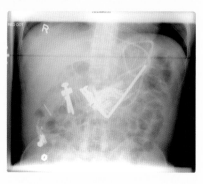 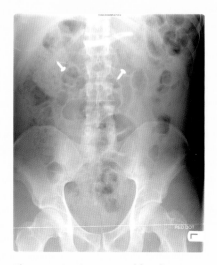

Figure 5.6d: Nuts and bolts   **Figure 5.6e: Screws and hook**

Case 7

A patient with right upper quadrant pain radiating to the right shoulder. Nausea and vomiting. High temperature. On examination the patient is tender in the right upper quadrant with guarding and a positive Murphy's sign.

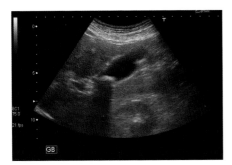

Figure 5.7a

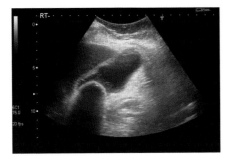

Figure 5.7b

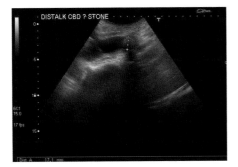

Figure 5.7c

Questions

Q1 What is the abnormality seen in these ultrasounds?

Q2 What is the most likely diagnosis and what are the features that allow you to make this diagnosis?

Q3 Which of Figures 5.7a and Figure 5.7b shows this?

Q4 What complications can occur?

Answers

(A1) Stones – within the gallbladder in Figures 5.7a and b and in the common bile duct (CBD) in Figure 5.7c.
The stones are hyperechoic with posterior acoustic shadowing.

(A2) Acute cholecystitis.
Distended gallbladder with a thickened wall (>3 mm), which is hard to delineate.
Halo sign – three-layered gallbladder wall with the middle layer being hypoechoic.

(A3) Figure 5.7b.

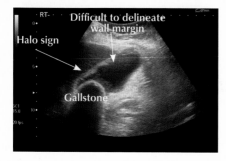

(A4) Abscess.
Mirizzi's syndrome.
Gangrene.
Emphysematous cholecystitis.
Bouveret's syndrome.
Gallstone ileus.
Empyema.

Case 8

A patient with abdominal pain and bowels not opening. On examination the abdomen is distended.

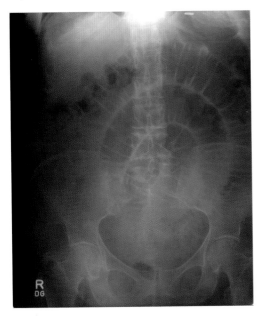

Figure 5.8a

Questions

(Q1) What abnormality is seen in the radiographs (Figures 5.8a and b) and what is the most likely diagnosis?

(Q2) Which is large bowel and which is small bowel? How can you tell?

(Q3) What are the causes in adults?

(Q4) What other imaging could be used?

(Q5) What complication is the main cause of concern, especially in Figure 5.8b?

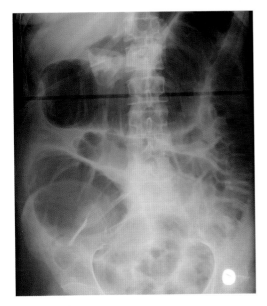

Figure 5.8b

Answers

(A1) Dilated loops of bowel, likely to be due to bowel obstruction.

(A2) Figure 5.8a shows dilated small bowel – the valvulae conniventes go completely across the bowel. The small bowel loops tend to lie together in a staircase pattern or in this case a spiral pattern.

Figure 5.8b shows dilated large bowel – the haustra pattern does not extend completely across the bowel, and the distended loops tend to be around the periphery along the expected location of the large bowel.

(A3) Adhesions.
Hernia.
Tumour.
Volvulus.
Intussusception.
Stone (gallstone ileus).

(A4) CT – look for a level of obstruction (cut-off point) and a possible cause, and for signs of perforation.

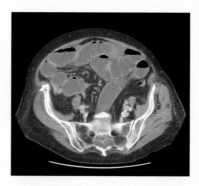

Figure 5.8c

(A5) Perforation due to the caecal pole being distended to >10 cm.

This image shows fluid-filled small-bowel loops, which are a sign of small-bowel obstruction.

These can be seen as a band of increased density (white arrow).

The obstruction is due to an inguinal hernia – seen here as gas in the right inguinal area.

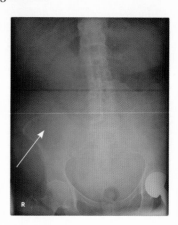

Figure 5.8d

Case 9

A patient with pain in the left flank radiating to the groin.

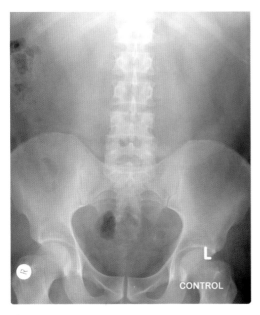

Figure 5.9a

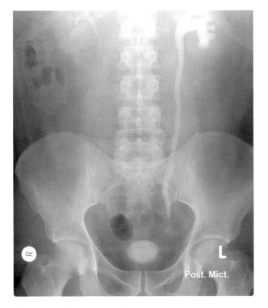

Figure 5.9b

Answers

(A1) Left-sided renal colic.

(A2) Intravenous urogram.

(A3) The control film shows a calculus within the left pelvis. The post-micturition film shows obstruction of the ureter with a standing column of contrast above the obstruction.

(A4) Yes – over 90% pass spontaneously.
Calculi < 4 mm pass in 90%.
Up to 8 mm in 50%.
Those over 8 mm rarely pass spontaneously and require treatment.

Case 10

A patient with left groin pain and night sweats, and raised inflammatory markers.

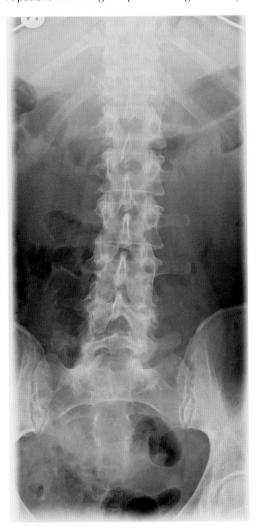

Figure 5.10a

Questions

Q1 What is the abnormality demonstrated in Figure 5.10a?

Q2 What is the most likely diagnosis?

Q3 What other type of imaging would be useful?

Answers

(A1) The right psoas shadow is bulging with a convex contour.

(A2) Right psoas abscess.

(A3) MRI.

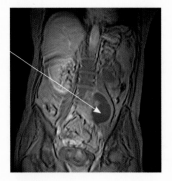

Figure 5.10b

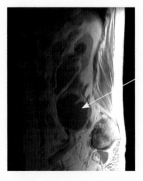

Figure 5.10c

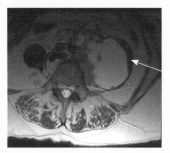

Figure 5.10d

Case 11

A patient complaining of acute pain radiating from the epigastrium to the back. Nausea and vomiting. High amylase in the blood.

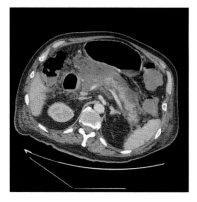

Figure 5.11

Questions

Q1   What is the likely diagnosis?

Q2   What are the signs of this on the CT (Figure 5.11)?

Q3   What are the clinical stages of this disease and which is this one?

Q4   What are common complications?

Q5   What are the treatment options for the different stages?

Answers

(A1) Pancreatitis.

(A2) Enlargement of pancreas with the margins becoming convex and ill-defined.
Stranding of surrounding fat, sparing the perirenal space (halo sign).
Heterogeneous parenchyma but mainly hypodense.
Non-enhancing portions of the pancreas – this indicates necrosis.
Not on this CT: hyperdensity in the pancreas indicates haemorrhagic pancreatitis.

(A3) I – oedematous pancreatitis.
II – partially necrotising pancreatitis.
III – totally necrotising pancreatitis.
This CT – II.

(A4) Phlegmon.
Pseudocyst.
Abscess.
Haemorrhagic pancreatitis.
Ascites.
Biliary obstruction.
Thrombosis of splenic vein and superior mesenteric vein.
Fistula.
Pseudoaneurysm.

(A5) I – conservative – 'drip and suck'.
Nasogastric tube, analgesic, prophylactic antibiotics.
II and III – surgery.

Case 12

A patient with haematuria and recurrent urinary infection.

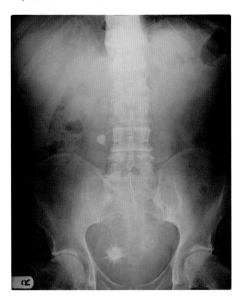

Figure 5.12a

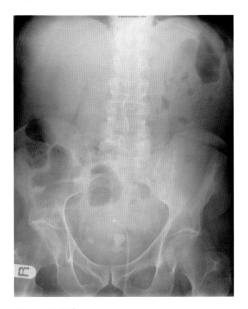

Figure 5.12b

Questions

(Q1)   What is the abnormality seen in both Figures 5.12a and b?

(Q2)   What are the different types?

(Q3)   If nothing is seen on the plain film does this rule out the diagnosis?

(Q4)   Are all types visible on radiology? If not, which ones are not?

(Q5)   Which are associated with infections?

(Q6)   Can they occur anywhere else in the urinary system?

(Q7)   How can they best be imaged?

Answers

(A1) Bladder stones seen within the pelvis.

(A2) Calcium stones.
Struvite stones.
Cystine stones.
Uric acid stones.
Xanthine stones.
Matrix stones.

(A3) NO – 30% are not seen. Some stones are radiolucent.

(A4) See above –
Struvite stones.
Uric acid stones.
Xanthine stones.
Matrix stones.

(A5) Struvite stones.
Matrix stones.

(A6) Yes – kidney and ureter.

(A7) Kidney – ultrasound.
Figure 5.12c shows a stone in the lower pole. It is echogenic with posterior acoustic shadowing.

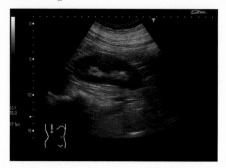

Figure 5.12c

Ureter – intravenous urogram – *see* Case 9.

Case 13

A patient with known ulcerative colitis presents with bloody profuse diarrhoea.

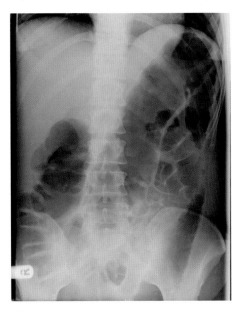

Figure 5.13a

Questions

(Q1) What is the most likely diagnosis?

(Q2) What features of this are shown in Figures 5.13a and b?

(Q3) What are the causes of this condition?

(Q4) What other imaging modality could be used?

(Q5) What is the prognosis?

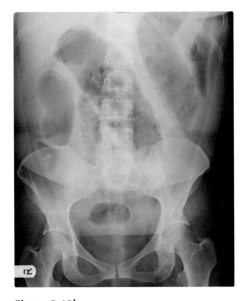

Figure 5.13b

Answers

(A1) Toxic megacolon.

(A2) Dilated loops of bowel with loss of haustra patterning.
Irregular mucosal surface.

(A3) Ulcerative colitis.
Crohn's disease.
Amoebiasis.
Salmonellosis.
Pseudomembranous colitis.
Ischaemic colitis.

(A4) CT.
NOT barium enema. This is contraindicated due to perforation risk.

(A5) Bad – 20% mortality rate.

Case 14

Victim of a road traffic collision.

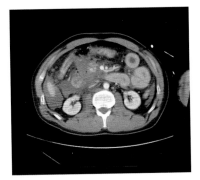

Figure 5.14a

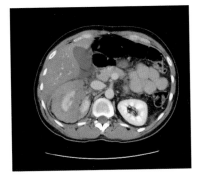

Figure 5.14b

Questions

Q1 What organs are involved in Figure 5.14a?

Q2 What organ is involved in Figure 5.14b?

Q3 What are the features in Figure 5.14a that indicate the patient is hypovolaemic?

Answers

(A1) The duodenum is ruptured.

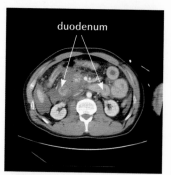

(A2) The right kidney is ruptured.

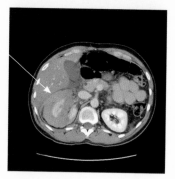

(A3) Collapsed IVC.
Shocked bowel:
- fluid filled, with thickened and enhanced bowel wall.

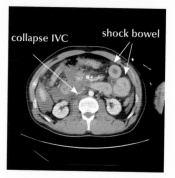

Reference

Dähnert W. *Radiology Review Manual.* 6th ed.
Philadelphia, PA: Lippincott Williams & Wilkins;
2007.

Index

Note: Question and Answer locators are given as Q/A.